MEANINGFUL USE

Jonathon L. Dreyer
Keith J. Dreyer, DO, PhD, FSIIM

A step-by-step approach to the Stage 1 CMS EHR Incentive Programs

Foreword by James H. Thrall, MD, FACR

" …To improve the quality of our health care while lowering its cost, we will make the immediate investments necessary to ensure that within five years, all of America's medical records are computerized. This will cut waste, eliminate red tape, and reduce the need to repeat expensive medical tests. But it just won't save billions of dollars and thousands of jobs—it will save lives by reducing the deadly but preventable medical errors that pervade our healthcare system… **"**

President Barack Obama
Speech on the Economy
George Mason University, Fairfax, VA
January 8, 2009

Contents

Foreword
By James H. Thrall, MD, FACR 9

Introduction 13

Part I:
The Fundamentals of Meaningful Use 19

Chapter 1
About the CMS EHR Incentive Programs 21

Chapter 2
Meaningful Use Legislation and Regulations 29

Chapter 3
Incentives and Penalties 39

Chapter 4
Meaningful Use Objectives and Measures 47

Chapter 5
Incentive Program Process Overview 63

Chapter 6
Product Certification 69

Chapter 7
Meaningful Use for Radiologists 91

Part II:
Building Your Strategy: 10 Steps to Achieving
Meaningful Use for Radiologists 101

Chapter 8
Preparing for Meaningful Use 103

Chapter 9
Developing Your Meaningful Use Strategy 117

Chapter 10
Executing Your Meaningful Use Strategy 131

Chapter 11
Sustaining Your Meaningful Use Strategy 143

Part III:
Imaging Provider Perspectives 155

Chapter 12
A Conversation with Dr. Keith J. Dreyer 157

Chapter 13
A Conversation with Dr. Alberto F. Goldszal 165

Chapter 14
A Conversation with Dr. David S. Mendelson 173

Chapter 15
A Conversation with Steven F. Fischer 181

Part IV:
Resources and Staying Informed 187

Chapter 16
Advocacy Efforts 189

Chapter 17
Resources and Important Dates 197

Chapter 18
Beyond Stage 1, Preparing for Stages 2 and 3 209

Chapter 19
Frequently Asked Questions for Radiologists 215

Chapter 20
Acronyms 225

Appendix 231

Sources 232

Index 234

Foreword

BY JAMES H. THRALL, MD, FACR

Each year, new terminology is added to the health care lexicon. One of the most important new terms for health care providers is the term *meaningful use* (MU). This term comes from the Health Information Technology for Economic and Clinical Health (HITECH) Act, the goal of which is to improve health care quality and safety and improve efficiency through promoting adoption of health information technology (HIT) and electronic health records (EHRs).

In order to promote the goals of the HITECH Act, the Centers for Medicare and Medicaid Services (CMS) have established financial incentive programs to encourage eligible professionals (EPs) and eligible hospitals (EHs) to adopt electronic health records. In order to judge whether professionals and eligible hospitals should receive the incentive payments, the concept of *meaningful use* of EHR technology was developed.

Jonathon L. Dreyer and Dr. Keith J. Dreyer have done a great service for radiologists in crafting their book entitled ***The Radiologist's Guide to Meaningful Use: A step-by-step approach to the Stage 1 CMS EHR Incentive Programs.*** They do a beautiful job in laying out the fundamental concepts underlying meaningful use—how meaningful use is defined and how the overall incentive program works.

The authors first help the individual reader understand whether and how he or she qualifies for the financial incentive program—it is estimated that more than 90 percent of radiologists will. For those eligible, this text lays out the pathway to success that radiologists will need to take in a systematic fashion to qualify for the meaningful use financial incentives and receive their share of the payments from CMS. They have done the heavy lifting and put potentially confusing regulations into logical and understandable terms including defining *meaningful use* itself.

The importance of the HITECH Act and its meaningful use financial incentive payments can be viewed both from the potential dollars involved and the likely secondary effects on radiology practices. From a purely financial standpoint the specialty-wide combination of potential payments and potential penalties for non-compliance is well over $1 billion in the aggregate and is likely to be in the range of hundreds of millions of dollars per year as the program matures toward the end of this decade. Individual radiologists can receive up to $44,000 over five years if they meet the program criteria and may be penalized if they do not.

Beyond the purely financial aspects, there will undoubtedly be non-financial implications. Patients will eventually become interested in knowing whether individual providers and hospitals have qualified for meaningful use under the HITECH Act. Providers and hospitals achieving success will be regarded as offering higher quality care and value than providers and institutions that fail to qualify. Therefore, it is in the interest of radiologists both financially and from the standpoint of practice development to understand meaningful use and take the appropriate steps to qualify for the financial incentive payments.

Jonathon and Keith Dreyer are to be congratulated for providing radiologists with a detailed road map to accomplish that important goal. ***The Radiologist's Guide to Meaningful Use*** should be immediately at hand in every radiology practice and department in the United States in order to maximize the likelihood of success and reduce uncertainty about meaningful use.

James H. Thrall, MD, FACR
Radiologist-in-Chief, Massachusetts General Hospital
Juan M. Taveras Professor of Radiology, Harvard Medical School

Introduction

With nearly $1.5 billion in available incentive payments for eligible diagnostic imaging professionals in the United States, each radiologist has the opportunity to receive up to $44,000 for achieving meaningful use before 2015. But in order to receive all incentive payments, meaningful use must begin by 2012. And starting in 2015, Medicare payment reductions will begin for not demonstrating meaningful use—hundreds of millions of dollars are at risk annually, and that number may reach billions if private payers start to mirror federal guidelines.

What is meaningful use?

Meaningful use, a term born out of the American Recovery and Reinvestment Act (ARRA) of 2009, refers to the use of certified electronic health record (EHR) technology to promote health care improvements and advance the electronic exchange of information among health care professionals. This program, designed to encourage health care professionals and hospitals to use certified EHR technology and demonstrate compliance through a series of measures and criteria, provides financial incentives for achieving health and efficiency goals over a prescribed timeframe.

Why did we create this guide?

Since the introduction of meaningful use, there has been miscommunication and confusion among medical specialists. In the radiology community, limited information and guidance has led to a number of meaningful use myths, including:

• Radiologists are not included in the CMS EHR Incentive Programs.

• Radiology was singled out of this government program.

• RIS, PACS, and other radiology IT solutions are excluded from meaningful use.

• Certain measures have been included or excluded from Stage 2 and/or 3.

• It is impossible for a radiologist to achieve meaningful use.

• Radiologists do not have to worry about penalties.

• If we wait, this will all go away.

All of the above statements are false. That's why we created this guide—to clear up the confusion, to provide a factual representation of the legislation and regulations as they apply to radiology professionals, and to offer a strategic approach to meaningful use for radiologists and the wider medical imaging community.

Who is this guide for?

Everyone involved in the management and delivery of diagnostic imaging services—ranging from radiologists to practice administrators, IT leads and CIOs, to healthcare IT vendors and others. This guide will help you prepare for meaningful use, develop and execute your strategy, and sustain your compliance with the CMS Electronic Health Records (EHR) Incentive Programs. While there are some chapters that will appeal more to one audience than another—for example, chapters 8–11 will be of particular interest to radiologists and practice administrators, while chapter 6 will be of particular interest to healthcare IT vendors—this guide provides a solid foundation for all medical imaging professionals interested in better understanding the CMS EHR Incentive Programs and being successful with meaningful use.

Inside this guide

This guide is divided into four parts and each section builds upon the prior to ensure you have the necessary tools to successfully achieve meaningful use in radiology.

- **Part I** covers the fundamentals of the CMS EHR Incentive Programs—providing an overview of the programs, legislation and regulation, incentives and penalties, objectives and measures, process overview, product certification guidelines, and how it all applies to radiologists.

- **Part II** provides a 10-step approach to becoming a meaningful user—preparing for meaningful use, developing your strategy, executing your strategy, and sustaining your meaningful use compliance.

- **Part III** examines how imaging practices are coping with meaningful use by interviewing leaders in the field—discussing their experiences and reviewing best practices for success.

- **Part IV** offers guidance for staying informed—discussing ongoing advocacy efforts, available resources and tools, important program dates, a brief look into the future, and FAQs for radiology professionals.

Online companion

Meaningful use is an evolving concept, and new information is always being published. This is far from a static topic. The companion website to this book, **theMUguide.com**, offers notification of content changes, information updates, and downloadable worksheets to be used in conjunction with this guide.

Companion worksheets

Many chapters point to worksheets that are designed to assist you in the planning, analysis, and compliance phase of your meaningful use strategy. These worksheets can be downloaded for free from **theMUguide.com**.

Quick Response (QR) codes and direct URLs

To enhance your experience, we have incorporated QR codes and direct URLs throughout the text of this guide. These codes will direct you to the online companion website where the most up-to-date information can be found. In order to use the QR codes, you will need a smartphone with a camera and QR code software. There are a number of free QR readers available, including Red Laser, QuickMark, and ScanLife, for multiple mobile device platforms.

Part I:
THE FUNDAMENTALS OF MEANINGFUL USE

In this section, we introduce the fundamentals of the CMS EHR Incentive Programs and review legislation, regulations, incentives and penalties, required objectives and measures, the meaningful use (MU) process, product certification requirements, and how this government program impacts the field of medical imaging. This material will provide you with a solid foundation as you prepare to develop your strategy for Stage 1 Meaningful Use and beyond.

CHAPTER 1
About the CMS EHR Incentive Programs

Get to know the basics.

Looking for even more information about the CMS EHR Incentive Programs? To access links to official program materials, documentation, and up-to-date information, scan the QR code above or go to **basics.theMUguide.com.**

In this chapter, we start you on your meaningful use (MU) journey and get you acquainted with the basics of the program—including how it all came about, the goals of MU, a high-level look at Stage 1 Meaningful Use requirements, and a brief glimpse of what's to come in Stages 2 and 3.

A five-year promise

On January 24, 2009, during his first Weekly Address as 44th president of the United States, President Barack Obama said that the nation's health records will be computerized within five years in order to lower health care costs, cut medical errors, and improve care.

In an effort to entice health care providers to jump onboard and begin to computerize their records, the government is incentivizing eligible physicians and hospitals under the Centers for Medicare and Medicaid Services (CMS) Electronic Health Records (EHR) Incentive Programs: paying up to $44,000 under Medicare and $63,750 under Medicaid. However, there is a catch. In order to qualify for this funding, provisions of the American Recovery and Reinvestment Act of 2009 and the Health Information Technology for Economic and Clinical Health (HITECH) Act require health care providers to show they are "meaningful users" of "certified" electronic health record systems over a specific timeline.

The road ahead

There is considerable pressure for all physicians, including specialists such as radiologists, to become meaningful users under the CMS EHR Incentive Programs. Determining provider eligibility, evaluating certified technology, and reviewing IT infrastructure are just a few of the necessary components for successful participation in these government programs. Meaningful use is moving rapidly, but the program is following a clear trajectory. Stage 1 Meaningful Use focuses on electronic data capture, while Stages 2 and 3 expand on this foundation by promoting quality, structured information exchange, safety, efficiency, and population health improvements.

The practice of medicine is changing, and EHR technology will undoubtedly provide medical providers with more information than ever before. Health care professionals will be able to access increased information about patients, share that information with colleagues at other facilities, and improve the quality of individual patients' care while monitoring and reporting data to federal committees to achieve health improvements for the population as a whole.

Goals of meaningful use

By focusing on the effective use of EHRs with certain capabilities, the HITECH Act makes it clear that the adoption of records is not a goal in itself: it is the use of EHRs to achieve health and efficiency goals that matters. HITECH's incentives and assistance programs seek to improve the health of Americans and the performance of their healthcare system through the meaningful use of EHRs to achieve five primary health care goals:

• Improve quality, safety, and efficiency while reducing health disparities.

• Engage patients and families in their health care.

• Promote and improve public and population health.

• Improve care coordination between providers.

• Ensure adequate privacy and security protections for personal health information.

In the context of the EHR Incentive Programs, demonstrating meaningful use is the key to receiving the incentive payments. It requires meeting a series of objectives that makes use of EHRs potential and is related to the improvement of quality, efficiency, and patient safety in the healthcare system through the use of certified technology.

Provider classification and eligibility

With the release of the final rule for Stage 1 Meaningful Use came a new definition to determine health care provider eligibility classification. Under the incentive programs, eligible hospital (EH) and eligible professional (EP) assignments are based on a series of CMS Place of Service (POS) Codes. The shift of POS 22 (outpatient hospital) from EH to EP, which came as a result of the Continuing Extension Act of 2010 (H.R. 4851), led to the majority of radiology professionals qualifying as EPs under the CMS EHR Incentive Programs. An outline of the place of service designation is below.

Eligible Hospital	*Eligible Professional*
POS 21: Inpatient Hospital	POS 11: Office
POS 23: Emergency Room	POS 20: Urgent Care Facility
	POS 22: Outpatient Hospital
	POS 24: Ambulatory Sx Center

Source: Centers for Medicare and Medicaid Services.

Based on this rule, most radiologists will qualify for meaningful use incentives and penalties unless they perform more than 90 percent of their services in the inpatient hospital (POS 21) or emergency room (POS 23) setting.

Two versions of the program

To further explain how these government programs impact radiologists, you need to understand that there are two versions of the CMS EHR Incentive Programs: one for Medicare providers and one for Medicaid providers. Under the Medicare EHR Incentive Program, EPs include doctors of medicine or osteopathy, doctors of dental surgery or dental medicine, doctors of podiatry, doctors of optometry, and chiropractors. Most radiologists fall under this classification.

For the Medicaid EHR Incentive Program, EPs include physicians (primarily doctors of medicine and doctors of osteopathy), nurse practitioners, certified nurse-midwives, dentists, and physician assistants who furnish services in a Federally Qualified Health Center or Rural Health Clinic that is led by a physician assistant.

The greatest distinctions between the two versions of the incentive programs are the financial upside and potential penalties. While the Medicare version offers up to $44,000 in incentives over five years per EP, the Medicaid version offers up to $63,750 per EP over six years. Furthermore, the Medicare program includes penalty adjustments, while there are no penalty adjustments under the Medicaid version of the CMS EHR Incentive Programs. Also, under Medicare, the meaningful use definition is common for all providers, while under Medicaid, states can adopt additional requirements for the program. Because the majority of radiologists applying for this program will fall under the EP and Medicare classification, this guide will focus on the Medicare version of the CMS EHR Incentive Programs for eligible professionals.

Stage 1 Meaningful Use

Capturing electronic health information and using that data to track and communicate clinical conditions is the predominant focus of Stage 1 Meaningful Use. Under both the Medicare and Medicaid versions of the incentive programs, the first phase of meaningful use includes measures that are specific to eligible hospitals (EHs) and eligible professionals (EPs). Radiologists, most of whom qualify as EPs under the Medicare version, have a total of 15 core set objectives, 10 menu set objectives, and 44 clinical quality measures (CQM) to report against. Each set has specific objectives that may be excluded, but all EPs are still required to "possess" EHR technology that has been tested and certified for all 33 Certification Criteria. In chapter 8, we review eligibility designation in detail, and in chapter 4, we discuss the core set, menu set, and clinical quality measures. Now let's take a brief look at an outline of the final measures for Stage 1 Meaningful Use.

15 Core Set Objectives and Measures

The 15 core set objectives and measures is required for all EPs. Six are eligible for exclusion. We discuss the core set objectives and measures in detail in chapter 4.

10 Menu Set Objectives and Measures

The 10 menu set objectives and measures allows EPs to select five of ten. Eight are eligible for exclusion. We discuss the menu set objectives and measures in detail in chapter 4.

44 Clinical Quality Measures (CQMs)

Clinical quality measures (CQMs) support health care processes, outcomes, patient perceptions, and organizational structures and provide CMS with the ability to assess how meaningful use and other programs are improving patient care. EPs are required to report three core or alternate core measures and three discretionary measures. We discuss the clinical quality measures in detail in chapter 4.

Stage 2 and Stage 3 Meaningful Use

In future rulemakings that will take place over the next few years, Stage 2 and Stage 3 of the government program will build on the foundation laid during Stage 1 Meaningful Use. In Stage 2, the medical community can expect to see an increased focus on Health Information Exchanges (HIEs), the mobilization of electronic health information across organizations within a region, community or health system, and electronic orders and results. Once successful, the program will continue in Stage 3 with an emphasis on quality, safety, and efficiency. This final stage of meaningful use will also promote decision support systems as well as patient access to self-management tools.

CHAPTER 2
Meaningful Use Legislation and Regulations

Learn more about the legislation and regulations.

To view the federal agency websites, committee documentation, and meeting schedules
and learn more about the laws and policies that shape these incentive programs, scan the
QR code above or go to **legislationandregulations.theMUguide.com.**

In this chapter, we examine the legislation and regulations that make up the CMS EHR Incentive Programs. We present a detailed, chronological account of the laws and policies that have shaped this government program. Understanding the history of the regulations offers insight as to where the program is headed.

The American Recovery and Reinvestment Act (ARRA) and Health Information and Technology for Economic and Clinical Health (HITECH) Act

It was more than two years ago that President Obama pledged a five year promise to computerize the nation's health records in an attempt to lower costs, cut medical errors, and improve patient care. A number of significant events have unfolded since this bold statement was made during his first Weekly Presidential Address.

In early 2009, just four days after he took office, Congress passed the American Recovery and Reinvestment (ARRA) Act of 2009, a $787 billion piece of legislation that now tops $840 billion, which President Obama quickly signed into law. Out of this new legislation came a sizable carve out: the Health Information and Technology for Economic and Clinical Health (HITECH) Act, designed to promote the adoption and meaningful use of health information technology. From this, roughly $20 billion was set aside to modernize healthcare IT systems through the CMS EHR Incentive Programs.

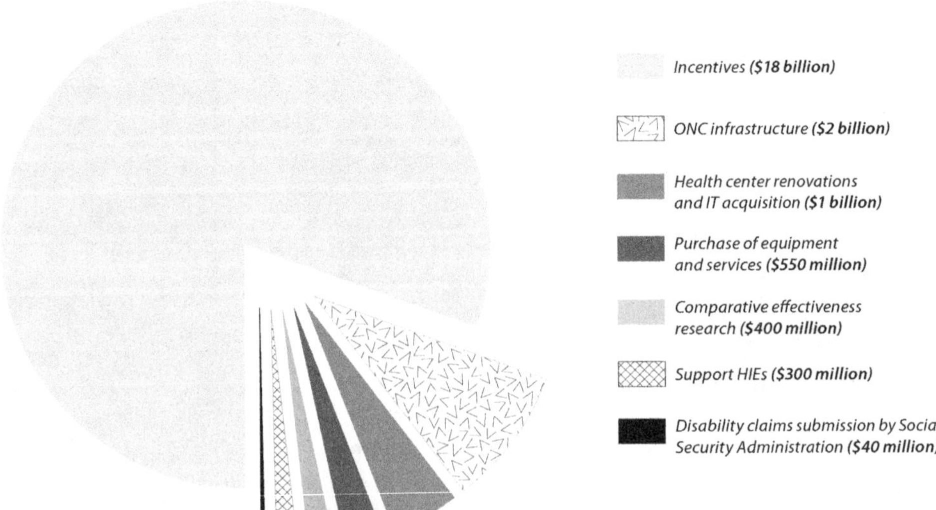

Shortly after being signed into law, a few significant developments unfolded, including:

• The Obama administration appointed David Blumenthal, MD, MPP, as National Coordinator for HIT at the Office of the National Coordinator (ONC).

• Under the auspices of the Federal Advisory Committee Act (FACA), two committees were formed: the Health IT Policy Committee (HITPC) and Health IT Standards Committee (HITSC).

• The American College of Radiology (ACR) proposed topics to the HIT Policy Committee that it viewed as relevant to the discussion of meaningful use for radiologists.

The Interim Final Rule (IFR) and Notice of Proposed Rulemaking (NPRM)

Just ten months after the introduction of the ARRA in 2009 and the HITECH Act, the ONC issued its Interim Final Rule (IFR), a summary of recommendations on meaningful use which proposed the initial set of standards and certification criteria as well as implementation specifications. At the same time, the Centers for Medicare and Medicaid Services (CMS) issued a Notice of Proposed Rulemaking (NPRM), which outlined three incentive programs and the provisions governing each program.

Following the release of the IFR and NPRM, a public comment period was initiated with a deadline of March 2010. In March 2010, the American College of Radiology (ACR), joined by the American Board of Radiology (ABR), Radiological Society of North America (RSNA), and Society for Imaging Informatics in Medicine (SIIM), issued a collective set of comments to all 25 reporting measures of the proposed EHR Incentive Programs as it applied to radiology.

Just one month later, in April 2010, the Continuing Extension Act of 2010 was passed—removing outpatient from the hospital-based definition of the legislation, and as a result, folding the majority of radiologists and other specialists into the mix.

CMS and ONC released the final rules of Stage 1 Meaningful Use in July 2010. In the months following the Final Rule issue, HHS announced the initial set of EHR testing and certification groups—Certification Commission for Health IT (CCHIT), Drummond Group (DGI), InfoGard Laboratories, ICSA Labs, SLI Global Solutions, and Surescripts. We discuss the role of these groups and the product certification process in chapter 6.

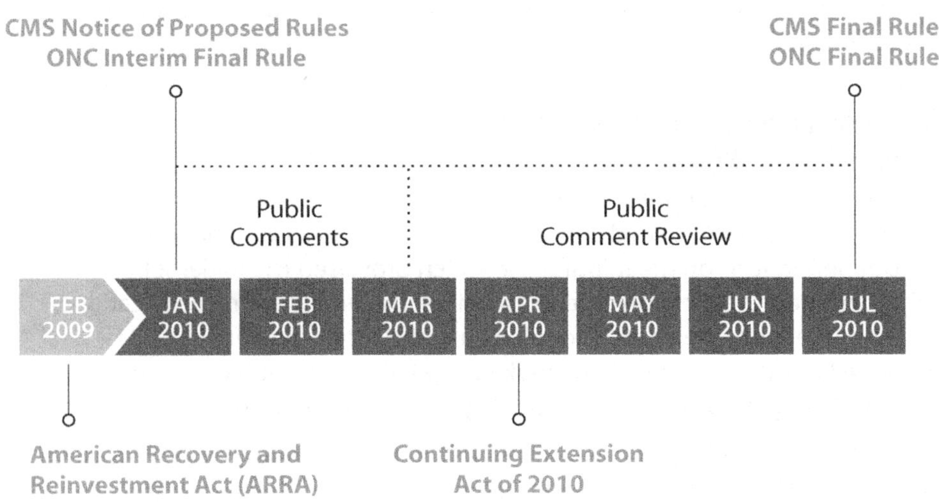

Comments from the radiology community

In early January 2011, the RSNA and ACR commented on the ONC RFI regarding the President's Council of Advisors on Science and Technology (PCAST) report. One month later, the ACR commented on the draft for Stage 2 Meaningful Use measure recommendations and verbally commented to the full HIT Policy Committee (HITPC) and MU Workgroup. Shortly thereafter, in April 2011, Dr. Farzad Mostashari was named the new National Coordinator for HIT at the ONC.

These significant events over the last few years have brought the medical community to where it is today with respect to this government program. Stage 1 Meaningful Use requirements and objectives are well established

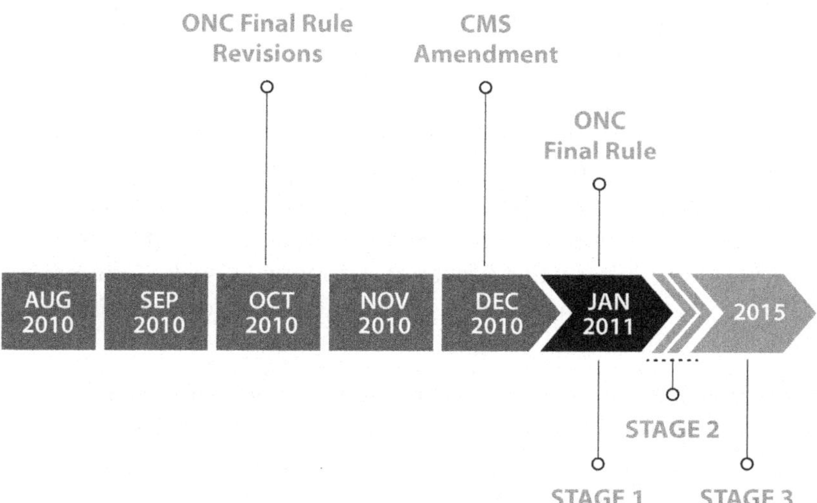

and clear, but the one-size-fits-all approach is not amenable to medical specialties. Despite this approach, medical specialists, including most radiologists, are eligible to participate and receive incentive payments and will ultimately be responsible for potential penalties starting in 2015.

Continued advocacy efforts by radiology societies will increase awareness, promote relevance, and help shape the requirements of future stages of the CMS EHR Incentive Programs. The expectation of these continued efforts is that future regulations will more closely reflect the goals and objectives that are relevant to medical specialists and their efforts for contributing to, and improving, patient care.

Two federal agencies working together

CMS and the ONC, both under the Department of Health and Human Services, hold joint responsibility for the development and implementation of the incentive programs. Under regulations of the HITECH Act, both federal agencies were initially responsible for creating a set of complementary final rules to support the implementation of the EHR Incentive Programs.

Moving forward, CMS continues to be responsible for regulating the "use" of technology by Medicare and Medicaid providers and the ONC holds responsibility for regulating the "technology" itself under regulations of the programs. Further, there are two advisory committees under the ONC, the HIT Policy Committee and HIT Standards Committee, with specific responsibilities related to meaningful use.

The HIT Policy Committee is responsible for providing recommendations to the ONC on the framework for development and adoption of a nationwide infrastructure, including standards for the exchange of patient medical information. Workgroups under this committee include: Meaningful Use, Certification/Adoption, Information Exchange, Nationwide Health Information Network (NHIN), Strategic Plan, Privacy & Security Policy, Enrollment, Privacy & Security Tiger Team, Governance, and Quality Measures.

The HIT Standards Committee is tasked with providing recommendations to the ONC on standards, implementation specifications, and certification criteria for the electronic exchange and use of health information. Workgroups under this committee include: Clinical Operations, Clinical Quality, Privacy & Security, Implementation, Vocabulary Task Force, and Power Team Summer Camp.

Stay Up-to-Date: Interested in learning more about the HIT Policy Committee and HIT Standards Committee? To view member details, upcoming meetings, past meetings, and workgroup recommendations or learn how to participate in meetings, scan the QR code at the beginning of this chapter or go to **legislationandregulation.theMUguide.com.**

For Stage 1 Meaningful Use, CMS has defined 25 objectives and measures to determine health care provider compliance and the ONC has defined 33 Certification Criteria to ensure technology provider software adheres to privacy, security, and functional criteria of the program. The following is an outline of the final regulations that were released by each federal agency.

CMS Final Rule: regulating use by providers

- Specifies initial criteria that eligible professionals (EPs), eligible hospitals (EHs), and critical access hospitals (CAHs) must meet to demonstrate meaningful use and qualify for incentive payments.

- Includes "core" criteria that all providers must meet to qualify for payments, while also allowing provider choice among a "menu set" of additional criteria.

- Outlines a phased approach to implement the requirements for demonstrating meaningful use. This approach initially establishes criteria for meaningful use based on currently available technological capabilities and providers' practice experience. CMS will establish graduated criteria for demonstrating meaningful use through future rulemaking, consistent with anticipated developments in technology and providers' capabilities.

ONC Final Rule: regulating technology

- Sets initial standards, implementation specifications, and certification criteria for EHR technology under the incentive program.

- Coordinates the standards required of EHR systems with the meaningful use requirements for eligible professionals and hospitals.

- With these standards in place, providers can be assured that the certified EHR technology they adopt is capable of performing the required functions to comply with CMS meaningful use requirements and other administrative requirements of the Medicare and Medicaid EHR Incentive Programs.

Meaningful use ascension path

According to a subcommittee report of the ONC HIT Policy Committee, meaningful use will follow an ascension path over time. In other words, each stage of meaningful use will affect subsequent stages through a multi-layered and interconnected approach to health care improvement. In effect, Stage 1 Meaningful Use forms the baseline of the program by promoting electronic data capture and information sharing. Stage 2 Meaningful Use focuses on advancing care processes, while Stage 3 Meaningful Use emphasizes leveraging the information collected in the first two stages to improve outcomes. Stages 2 and 3 both build on the foundation of Stage 1 Meaningful Use and will be developed over the next few years through a series of future rulemakings.

CHAPTER 3
Incentives and Penalties

Find out even more about the incentives and penalties.

To discover additional program opportunities, learn more about payment specifications, download incentive and penalty tables, review the list of HPSAs, and more, scan the QR code above or go to **incentivesandpenalties.theMUguide.com.**

In this chapter, we look at the incentive opportunities as well as the program penalties for non-compliance. We also discuss additional financial benefits for providers that meet certain criteria and introduce a few details about how payments are issued for demonstrating meaningful use.

Up to $44,000 per eligible radiologist

All eligible professionals (EPs) have an opportunity to receive up to $44,000 in incentive payments through the Medicare EHR Incentive Program based on year of participation (see payment table). Under the Medicaid EHR Incentive Program, EPs have the potential to receive up to $63,750 over a six-year period. In chapter 1, we explained how most radiologists qualify as EPs under the Medicare EHR Incentive Program. As a result of this classification, the majority of U.S.-based radiologists will qualify for meaningful use incentives and penalties.

Meaningful use program incentives

Incentive payments are based on calendar year and the reporting period for the first year is any ninety continuous days during the calendar year. For years 2011–2016, eligible professionals who demonstrate meaningful use of certified EHR technology can receive up to $44,000 over the duration of the Medicare program (ninety-day reporting period must begin by October 3, 2012 in order to receive the full incentive opportunity). The following table outlines the incentive opportunities for a Medicare EP.

MAXIMUM PAYMENT UNDER MEDICARE EHR INCENTIVE PROGRAM

Calendar Year	2011	2012	2013	2014	2015+
2011	Up to $18,000	—	—	—	$0
2012	Up to $12,000	Up to $18,000	—	—	$0
2013	Up to $8,000	Up to $12,000	Up to $15,000	—	$0
2014	Up to $4,000	Up to $8,000	Up to $12,000	Up to $12,000	$0
2015	Up to $2,000	Up to $4,000	Up to $8,000	Up to $8,000	$0
2016	—	Up to $2,000	Up to $4,000	Up to $4,000	$0
Total	**Up to $44,000**	**Up to $44,000**	**Up to $39,000**	**Up to $24,000**	**$0**

Source: Centers for Medicare and Medicaid Services.

Note: Incentives cannot exceed 75 percent of an EP's total Medicare Physician Fee Schedule compensation for any given year. For 2011/2012, an EP would need to have at least $24,000 in allowed Medicare Physician Fee Schedule charges in order to reap the full $18,000 year one incentive payment ($18,000 being 75 percent of $24,000). Keep in mind that the threshold for allowed charges in subsequent years will vary based on the amount of the incentive opportunity.

In addition to the potential incentive payments outlined above, EPs that predominantly furnish services (more than 50 percent) in a designated Health Professional Shortage Area (HPSA) may qualify for an additional 10 percent bonus payment for each year of successful program participation.

HPSAs are designated by the U.S. Department of Health and Health Resources and Services Administration (HRSA) as having shortages of primary medical care, dental, or mental health providers and may be geographic (a county or service area), demographic (low income population), or institutional (comprehensive health center, federally qualified health center, or other public facility). Medically Underserved Areas/Populations are areas or populations designated by HRSA as having: (1) too few primary care providers, (2) high infant mortality, (3) high poverty, and/or (4) high elderly population. At the time of writing, there were more than six thousand HPSAs with sixty-five million people living in them.

Stay Up-to-Date: Not sure if you are eligible for an incentive bonus payment? To read more about HPSAs, and to identify if you may qualify to receive additional incentives for each year of successful program participation, scan the QR code at the beginning of this chapter or go to **incentivesandpenalties.theMUguide.com.**

Meaningful use program penalties

Under the Medicare version of the program, payment adjustments go into effect beginning in 2015 if an EP does not successfully demonstrate meaningful use of certified EHR technology. The non-trivial penalties are outlined in the table below. For EPs, including radiologists, this comes in the form of an adjustment to the physician fee schedule amount for covered professional services.

POTENTIAL PAYMENT REDUCTIONS UNDER MEDICARE EHR INCENTIVE PROGRAM

Calendar Year	*Payment Reductions*
2015	Minus 1% of total Medicare fee schedule compensation
2016	Minus 2% of total Medicare fee schedule compensation
2017	Minus 3% of total Medicare fee schedule compensation
2018	Minus 3%, or minus 4% if >75% of EPs are not demonstrating meaningful use
2019+	Minus 3%, or minus 5% if >75% of EPs are not demonstrating meaningful use

Source: Centers for Medicare and Medicaid Services.

So, if you are eligible for the CMS EHR Incentive Programs and you do not successfully demonstrate meaningful use of certified EHR technology by 2015 (for Medicare EPs), you will be subject to payment adjustments of your Medicare reimbursement. Payment reductions will start at 1 percent and will increase each year that EPs do not demonstrate meaningful use (up to a maximum of 5 percent).

The final legislation allows for annual hardship exemptions on a case-by-case basis. If applicable, this exemption could relieve certain EPs from the impending payment adjustments for up to five years. More information about hardship exemptions will be provided in future rulemaking prior to 2015.

If the medical imaging community fails to comply with meaningful use criteria, hundreds of millions of dollars may be at risk every year, and that could easily reach billions if private payers begin to adopt guidelines that mirror federal policy.

Meaningful use incentive payments

Once your imaging practice has determined your participation eligibility, and prior to receiving incentive payments, each EP will need to: (1) obtain a National Provider Identifier, (2) enroll in the CMS Provider Enrollment Chain and Ownership System, and (3) have an active account in the National Plan and Provider Enumeration System. Details about these requirements can be found on the CMS EHR Incentive Programs website. We will discuss the entire process in chapter 11.

Once an EP meets the requirements prescribed in the Medicare version of the program, they will have to demonstrate meaningful use through the CMS web-based Registration and Attestation System. In this system, health care providers will enter their numerators and denominators for each core set, menu set, and clinical quality measure discussed in the next chapter. Additionally, EPs will use this system to legally attest that they have successfully demonstrated meaningful use.

Upon successfully demonstrating meaningful use and attesting, EPs, including eligible radiologists, participating in the Medicare version of the incentive program will receive a single lump sum payment for each year that they continue to demonstrate meaningful use of certified EHR technology for a total incentive payment of up to $44,000 over five consecutive years. If an EP provides service in an HPSA, the additional payment bonus will be paid separately on an annual basis.

Note: The American Recovery and Reinvestment Act of 2009 requires that CMS post the names, business addresses, and business phone numbers of all Medicare eligible professionals and hospitals who receive EHR Incentive Payments.

The opportunity is significant. In fact, during the first year of this program, the government issued approximately $1 billion in incentive payments to EPs and EHs that successfully demonstrated meaningful use.

CHAPTER 4
Meaningful Use Objectives and Measures

Read more about the objectives and measures.

To review core set, menu set, and clinical quality measures online, obtain access
to program updates, and review specifications related to radiology EPs, scan the
QR code above or go to **objectivesandmeasures.theMUguide.com.**

In this chapter, we discuss the objectives and measures that make it possible to assess the effectiveness of the incentive programs. We take a look at the core set, menu set, and clinical quality measures that must be reported by EPs participating in the program. We also brush the surface on exclusion opportunities that are discussed at greater lengths in chapter 8.

Core, Menu, and Clinical Quality Measures

Capturing electronic health information and using that data to track and communicate clinical conditions is the predominant focus of Stage 1 Meaningful Use. This first phase of meaningful use includes measures that are specific to EHs and EPs. Radiology EPs have a total of 15 core set objectives, 10 menu set objectives, and 44 clinical quality measures to report against. Each set has specific objectives that may be excluded. However, all EPs are still required to "possess" EHR technology that has been tested and certified against all 33 Certification Criteria.

CMS has relaxed the requirements for 2011 and 2012 in response to public comments. An outline of the final measures for Stage 1 Meaningful Use is below.

15 Core Set Measures: The core set includes six measures eligible for exclusion. For radiology EPs, three of the measures may potentially be excluded based on practice type and patient population. Of the remaining objectives, eight may be achievable with your current IT investments while the remaining measure will likely require your department to implement new, certified technology modules.

10 Menu Set Measures: The menu set includes eight measures eligible for exclusion and allows EPs to select five of 10 measures to report. For radiology EPs, three measures may potentially be excluded based on practice type and patient population. Based on menu set requirements, most radiology EPs would be responsible for reporting two of seven menu set measures. Like the core set measures, menu set measures will likely require implementation of new certified technology in order to comply with meaningful use objectives.

44 Clinical Quality Measures (CQMs): One of the core set objectives, 42 CFR §495.6(d)(10), expands out to a set of 44 clinically based measures of which EPs are required to report on six (three core or alternate core measures and three discretionary measures).

Core Set Objectives and Measures

Satisfying the requirements of the Medicare EHR Incentive Program is determined by compliance with a variety of meaningful use measures. All EPs are required to report the following 15 core set measures except when exclusion criteria are met.

CORE SET OBJECTIVES AND MEASURES

Objective	Measure	Exclusion
42 CFR §495.6(d)(1) Use computerized provider order entry (CPOE) for medication orders directly entered by any licensed health care professional who can enter orders into the medical record per state, local, and professional guidelines	More than 30% of unique patients with at least one medication in their medication list seen by the EP have at least one medication order entered using CPOE	Any EP who writes fewer than 100 prescriptions during the EHR reporting period
42 CFR §495.6(d)(2) Implement drug-drug and drug-allergy interaction checks	The EP has enabled this functionality for the entire EHR reporting period	N/A
42 CFR §495.6(d)(3) Maintain an up-to-date problem list of current and active diagnoses	More than 80% of all unique patients seen by the EP have at least one entry or an indication that no problems are known for the patient recorded as structured data	N/A
42 CFR §495.6(d)(4) Generate and transmit permissible prescriptions electronically (eRx)	More than 40% of all permissible prescriptions written by the EP are transmitted electronically using certified EHR technology	Any EP who writes fewer than 100 prescriptions during the EHR reporting period
42 CFR §495.6(d)(5) Maintain active medication list	More than 80% of all unique patients seen by the EP have at least one entry (or an indication that the patient is not currently prescribed any medication) recorded as structured data	N/A

Objective	Measure	Exclusion
42 CFR §495.6(d)(6) Maintain active medication allergy list	More than 80% of all unique patients seen by the EP have at least one entry (or an indication that the patient has no known medication allergies) recorded as structured data	N/A
42 CFR §495.6(d)(7) Record demographics: preferred language, gender, race, ethnicity, date of birth	More than 50% of all unique patients seen by the EP have demographics recorded as structured data	N/A
42 CFR §495.6(d)(8) Record and chart changes in vital signs: height, weight, blood pressure. Calculate and display BMI, plot and display growth charts for children 2–20 years (including BMI)	More than 50% of all unique patients age 2 and over seen by the EP have height, weight, and blood pressure recorded as structured data	Any EP who either sees no patients 2 years or older, or who believes that all three vital signs of height, weight, and blood pressure of their patients have no relevance in their scope of practice
42 CFR §495.6(d)(9) Record smoking status for patients 13 years old or older	More than 50% of all unique patients 13 years old or older seen by the EP have smoking status recorded as structured data	Any EP who sees no patients 13 years and older
42 CFR §495.6(d)(10) Report ambulatory clinical quality measures to CMS or the States	For 2011, provide aggregate numerator and denominator, and exclusions through attestation as required by CMS and for 2012, electronically submit the CQMs as required by CMS	N/A
42 CFR §495.6(d)(11) Implement one clinical decision support rule relevant to specialty or high clinical priority along with the ability to track compliance with that rule	Implement one clinical decision support rule	N/A

Objective	Measure	Exclusion
42 CFR §495.6(d)(12) Provide patients with an electronic copy of their health information (including diagnostic test results, problem list, medication lists, medication allergies) upon request	More than 50% of all patients who request an electronic copy of their health information are provided it within three business days	Any EP that has no requests from patients or their agents for an electronic copy of patient health information during the EHR reporting period
42 CFR §495.6(d)(13) Provide clinical summaries for patients for each office visit	Clinical summaries provided to patients for more than 50% of all office visits within three business days	Any EP who has no office visits during the EHR reporting period
42 CFR §495.6(d)(14) Capability to exchange key clinical information (for example: problem list, medication list, medication allergies, diagnostic test results) among providers of care and patient authorized entities electronically	Performed at least one test of certified EHR technology's capacity to electronically exchange key clinical information	N/A
42 CFR §495.6(d)(15) Protect electronic health information created or maintained by the certified EHR technology through the implementation of appropriate technical capabilities	Conduct or review a security risk analysis per 45 CFR 164.308 (a)(1) and implement security updates as necessary and correct identified security deficiencies as part of its risk management process	N/A

Source: Centers for Medicare and Medicaid Services.

Core Set and Radiology

Due to the one-size-fits-all approach of the government incentive programs, radiology practices will need to adapt some of the core set requirements and acquire new data points to satisfy program requirements. Despite these core objectives and measures that do not perfectly align with typical radiology activities, exclusion opportunities do exist. In chapter 8, we provide details about how to conduct an exemption analysis to determine potential core set exclusion opportunities, thus reducing your requirements for data capture and reporting.

Even though the regulations are not geared toward radiologists, you should look at the positive. In addition to the incentive payments, your imaging practice should seek other benefits of the program—better data structure, better practice management capabilities, and better information that can be preserved in your IT systems.

Menu Set Objectives and Measures

Satisfying the requirements of the Medicare EHR Incentive Program is determined by compliance with a variety of additional measures beyond the core set. All EPs are required to report five of the following 10 menu set measures except when exclusion criteria are met. If an EP meets the exclusion criteria for one menu set measure, they would select four of the remaining nine measures; if an EP meets exclusion criteria for two menu set measures, they would select three of the remaining eight; if an EP meets exclusion criteria for three menu set measures, they would select two of the remaining seven; and so on.

MENU SET OBJECTIVES AND MEASURES

Objective	Measure	Exclusion
42 CFR §495.6(e)(1) Implement drug-formulary checks	The EP has enabled this functionality and has access to at least one internal or external formulary for the entire EHR reporting period	Any EP who writes fewer than 100 prescriptions during the EHR reporting period
42 CFR §495.6(e)(2) Incorporate clinical lab test results into certified EHR technology as structured data	More than 40% of all clinical lab test results ordered by the EP during the EHR reporting period whose results are either in a positive/negative or numerical format are incorporated in certified EHR technology as structured data	An EP who orders no lab tests whose results are either in a positive/negative or numeric format during the EHR reporting period
42 CFR §495.6(e)(3) Generate lists of patients by specific conditions to use for quality improvement, reduction of disparities, research, or outreach	Generate at least one report listing patients of the EP with a specific condition	N/A
42 CFR §495.6(e)(4) Send reminders to patients per patient preference for preventive/follow-up care	More than 20% of all unique patients 65 years or older or 5 years old or younger were sent an appropriate reminder during the EHR reporting period	An EP who has no patients 65 years or older or 5 years old or younger with records maintained using certified EHR technology
42 CFR §495.6(e)(5) Provide patients with timely electronic access to their health information (including lab results, problem list, medication lists, medication allergies) within four business days of the information being available to the EP	More than 10% of all unique patients seen by the EP are provided timely (available to the patient within four business days of being updated in the certified EHR technology) electronic access to their health information subject to the EP's discretion to withhold certain information	Any EP that neither orders nor creates any of the information listed at 45 CFR 170.304(g) during the EHR reporting period

Objective	Measure	Exclusion
42 CFR §495.6(e)(6) Use certified EHR technology to identify patient-specific education resources and provide those resources to the patient if appropriate	More than 10% of all unique patients seen by the EP during the EHR reporting period are provided patient-specific education resources	N/A
42 CFR §495.6(e)(7) The EP who receives a patient from another setting of care or provider of care or believes an encounter is relevant should perform medication reconciliation	The EP performs medication reconciliation for more than 50% of transitions of care in which the patient is transitioned into the care of the EP	An EP who was not the recipient of any transitions of care during the reporting period
42 CFR §495.6(e)(8) The EP who transitions their patient to another setting of care or refers their patient to another provider of care should provide summary of care record for each transition of care or referral	The EP who transitions their patient to another setting of care or provider of care provides a summary of care record for more than 50% of transitions of care and referrals	An EP who neither transfers a patient to another setting nor refers a patient to another provider during the EHR reporting period

Objective	Measure	Exclusion
42 CFR §495.6(e)(9) Capability to submit electronic data to immunization registries or Immunization Information Systems and actual submission in accordance with applicable law and practice	Performed at least one test of certified EHR technology's capacity to submit electronic data to immunization registries and follow up submission if the test is successful (unless none of the immunization registries to which the EP submits such information have the capacity to receive the information electronically)	An EP who administers no immunizations during the EHR reporting period or where no immunization registry has the capacity to receive the information electronically
42 CFR §495.6(e)(10) Capability to submit electronic syndromic surveillance data to public health agencies and actual submission in accordance with applicable law and practice	Performed at least one test of certified EHR technology's capacity to provide electronic syndromic surveillance data to public health agencies and follow-up submission if the test is successful (unless none of the public health agencies to which an EP submits such information have the capacity to receive the information electronically)	An EP who does not collect any reportable syndromic information on their patients during the EHR reporting period or does not submit such information to any public health agency that has the capacity to receive the information electronically

Source: Centers for Medicare and Medicaid Services.

Menu Set and Radiology

As with the core set, radiology practices will need to adapt some of the menu set requirements and acquire new data points to satisfy program requirements. The menu set offers a greater opportunity for exclusions and more flexibility for radiology professionals than the core set. Similar to the core set, in chapter 8 we provide details about how to conduct an exemption analysis to determine potential menu set exclusion opportunities.

Note: Unless an EP has an exception for all menu set objectives and measures, they must complete at least one of the Public Health measures (Capability to submit electronic data to immunization registries or Immunization Information Systems and actual submission in accordance with applicable law and practice -or- Capability to submit electronic syndromic surveillance data to public health agencies and actual submission in accordance with applicable law and practice) as part of their demonstration of the menu set in order to be a meaningful user of certified EHR technology.

Clinical Quality Measures (CQMs)

To meet program requirements and successfully demonstrate meaningful use, EPs are required to report clinical quality measures in addition to the core set and menu set measures. EPs only have to demonstrate a total of six of the 44 clinical quality measures: three core/alternate core measures and three discretionary measures from the remaining 38 measures.

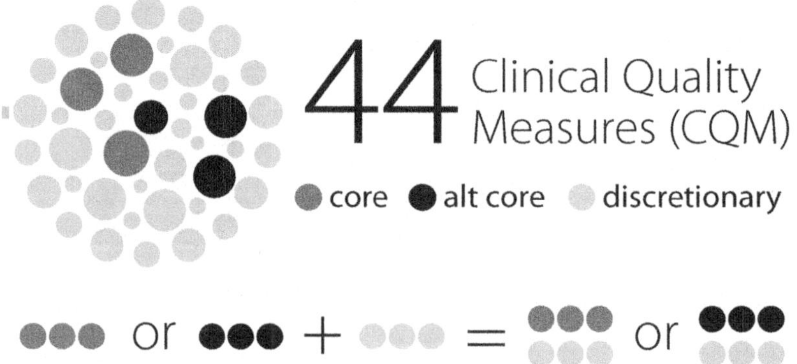

There are percentage-based measures that require the collection of numerator and denominator information to calculate and determine if minimum thresholds are met. If an EP has a denominator of zero for all core and alternate core measures, they could comply by reporting zeros. It is important to note that EPs must report this information even if they have no patients in the denominator.

CQM Core Set **(3 - Cardiac, Tobacco, Obesity)**	**CQM Alternate Set** **(3 - Obesity, Immunizations)**
• Hypertension blood pressure measurement (NQF 0013) • Tobacco use assessment and cessation intervention (NQF 0028) • Adult weight screening and follow-up (NQF 0421, PQRI 128)	• Weight assessment and counseling for children and adolescents (NQF 0024) • Influenza immunization for patients 50 or older (NQF 0041, PQRI 110) • Childhood immunization status (NQF 0038)

CQM Menu Set – Cardiac (10 of 38 discretionary measures)

• Heart failure: ACE Inhibitor or ARB therapy for LVSD (NQF 0081, PQRI 5)

• Heart failure: Warfarin therapy patients with atrial fibrillation (NQF 0084, PQRI 200)

• Heart failure: Beta-blocker therapy for LVSD (NQF 0083, PQRI 8)

• CAD: Beta-blocker therapy for CAD patients with prior Myocardial Infarction (MI) (NQF 0070, PQRI 7)

• CAD: Drug therapy for lowering LDL-Cholesterol (NQF 0074, PQRI 197)

• CAD: Oral antiplatelet therapy prescribed for CAD patients (NQF0061, PQRI 6)

• Ischemic vascular disease: Blood pressure management (NQF 0073, PQRI 201)

• Ischemic vascular disease: Use of aspirin or other antithrombotic (NQF 0068, PQRI 204)

• Ischemic vascular disease: Complete lipid panel and LDL control (NQF 0075)

• Controlling high blood pressure (NQF 0018)

CQM Menu Set – Diabetes (9 of 38 discretionary measures)

• Diabetes: Hemoglobin A1c poor control (NQF 0059, PQRI 1)

• Diabetes: Low Density Lipoprotein (LDL) management and control (NQF 0064, PQRI 2)

• Diabetes: Blood pressure management (NQF 0061, PQRI 3)

• Diabetes: Hemoglobin A1c control (less than 8.0%) (NQF 0575)

• Diabetes: Eye exam (NQF 0055, PQRI 117)

• Diabetes: Urine screening (NQF 0062, PQRI 119)

• Diabetes: Foot exam (NQF 0056, PQRI 163)

• Diabetic retinopathy: Presence of macular edema and retinopathy severity (NQF 0088, PQRI 18)

• Diabetic retinopathy: Communication with physician managing ongoing care (NQF 0089, PQRI 19)

CQM Menu Set – Oncology (6 of 38 discretionary measures)

- Breast cancer screening (NQF 0031, PQRI 112)
- Breast cancer: Hormonal therapy for Stage IC-IIIC Estrogen receptor positive (NQF 0387, PQRI 71)
- Colorectal cancer screening (NQF 0034, PQRI 113)
- Colon cancer: Chemotherapy for Stage III patients (NQF 0385, PQRI 72)
- Cervical cancer screening (NQF 0032)
- Prostate cancer: Avoidance of bone scan overuse for staging low-risk cancer (NQF 0389, PQRI 102)

CQM Menu Set – Asthma (3 of 38 discretionary measures)

- Asthma pharmacologic therapy (NQF 0047, PQRI 53)
- Asthma assessment (NQF 0001, PQRI 64)
- Use of appropriate medications for asthma (NQF 0036)

CQM Menu Set – Infections (3 of 38 discretionary measures)

- Chlamydia screening for women (NQF 0033)
- Pneumonia vaccine status of their patients (NQF 0043, PQRI 111)
- Testing for children with pharyngitis (NQF 0002, PQRI 66)

CQM Menu Set – Dependencies (3 of 38 discretionary measures)

- Smoking and tobacco use cessation: Counseling for cessation strategies (NQF 0027, PQRI 115)
- Initiation and engagement of alcohol and other drug dependence treatments (NQF 0004)
- Antidepressant medication management (NQF 0105, PQRI 9)

CQM Menu Set – Prenatal Care (2 of 38 discretionary measures)

- Prenatal care: Screening for HIV (NQF 0012)
- Prenatal care: Anti-D Immune Globulin (NQF 0014)

CQM Menu Set – Glaucoma (1 of 38 discretionary measures)

- Primary open angle glaucoma (POAG): Optic nerve evaluation (NQF 0086, PQRI 12)

CQM Menu Set – Low Back Pain (1 of 38 discretionary measures)

- Appropriate use of imaging studies (NQF 0052)

CQMs and Radiology

As with the core set and menu set measures, there are certain CQMs that are more likely to be relevant to diagnostic imaging professionals than others. As you will recall, EPs are required to select three core/alternate core CQMs in addition to three selections from the discretionary set. If an EP reports zeros for one or more of the required core CQMs, they must then report on up to three alternate core CQMs.

The following three core CQMs will be selected by most radiology EPs.

- **NFQ 0013 – Hypertension Blood Pressure Measurement:** Percentage of patient visits for patients aged 18 years and older with a diagnosis of hypertension who have been seen for at least 2 office visits, with blood pressure (BP) recorded.

- **NQF 0028 – Tobacco Use Assessment and Cessation Intervention:** (a) Percentage of patients aged 18 years or older who have been seen for at least 2 office visits, who were queried about tobacco use one or more times within 24 months. (b) Percentage of patients aged 18 years and older identified as tobacco users within the past 24 months and have been seen for at least 2 office visits, who received cessation intervention.

- **NQF 0421/PQRI 128 – Adult Weight Screening and Follow-up:** Percentage of patients aged 18 years and older with a calculated BMI in the past six months or during the current visit documented in the medical record and if the most recent BMI is outside parameters, a follow-up plan is documented.

The following discretionary measures are examples of CQMs that are not only easier to capture as a result of their yes/no format, but also provide the most value from a clinical information standpoint for radiology EPs.

- **NFQ 0043/PQRI 111 – Pneumonia Vaccination Status for Older Adults:** Percentage of patients 65 years of age and older who have ever received pneumococcal vaccine.

- **NQF 0031/PQRI 112 – Breast Cancer Screening:** Percentage of women 40–69 years of age who had a mammogram to screen for breast cancer.

- **NQF 0034/PQRI 113 – Colorectal Cancer Screening:** Percentage of adults 50–75 years of age who had appropriate screening for colorectal cancer.

The examples above are simply suggestions. The CQMs for your radiology EPs may vary based on practice setting, workflow, and available technology. In chapter 6, we discuss product certification steps that your healthcare IT vendors must undertake if you anticipate using their technology as part of your meaningful use strategy.

4

CHAPTER 5
Incentive Program Process Overview

Understand how it all fits together.

Meaningful use involves a series of complex interactions between various government agencies, healthcare IT providers, and health care professionals. To learn more about how it all fits together, scan the QR code above or go to **process.theMUguide.com.**

In this chapter, we examine the interactions that take place between federal agencies, medical professionals, and IT providers. Understanding how these groups interact and fit together is critical to truly understanding the ins and outs of the CMS EHR Incentive Programs.

Meaningful use process overview

We have already discussed how meaningful use is a joint effort shared by the Office of the National Coordinator for Health IT (ONC) and the Centers for Medicare and Medicaid Services (CMS), both operating under the Department of Health and Human Services (HHS). In chapter 2, we also reviewed how the ONC regulates the "technology" and how CMS regulates the "professionals." Now let's take a look at a high-level overview of the process and how these agencies relate to healthcare IT providers, health care professionals, and the incentive payments under this government program.

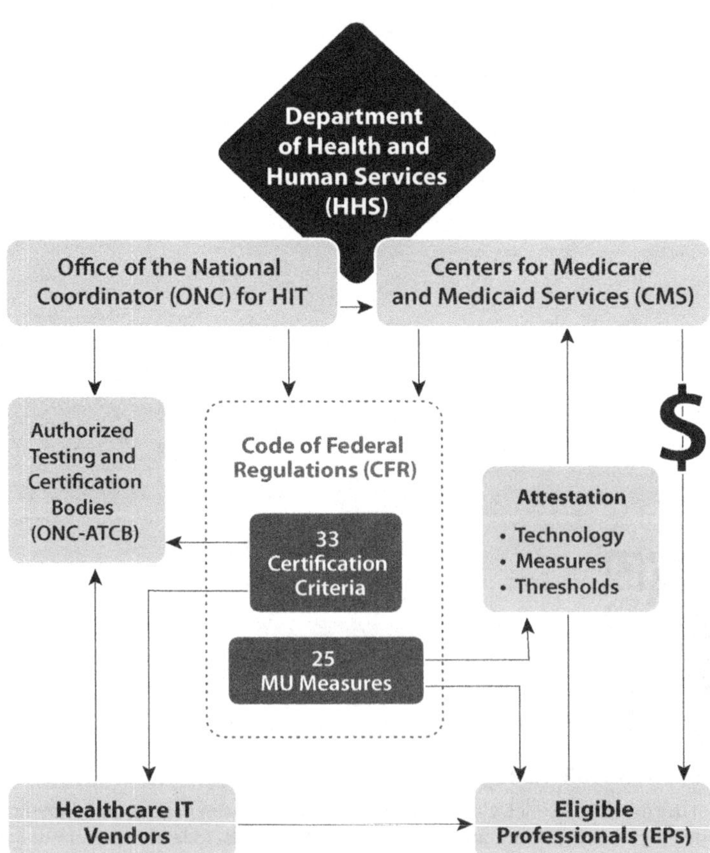

For Stage 1 Meaningful Use, the regulations were passed and both 25 meaningful use measures and 33 Certification Criteria were entered into the Code of Federal Regulations (CFR). The 33 Certification Criteria are what vendors, or health care providers with their own in-house developed EHR technology, review to make sure that their products are compliant with the program. The 25 meaningful use measures are what EPs review to make sure that they are compliant with all applicable objectives and measures.

Further, the ONC has authorized non-federal agencies in the private sector to test and certify healthcare IT products to ensure they are compliant with meaningful use. Vendors, or health care providers with their in-house developed EHR technology, will submit their technology to an authorized agency (an ONC-ATCB) to gain either modular or complete certification. Once certified, products can be made available to the EP community for use in the CMS EHR Incentive Programs. In chapter 6, we discuss the product certification process in detail.

Once an EP has selected, implemented, and begun using certified EHR technology to demonstrate meaningful use, all EPs are required to attest to CMS regarding their compliance with all objectives and their associated measures. After an EP has satisfied all required measures, including the notation of exclusions, and meets minimum program thresholds, incentive payments will be made by CMS. Payments are made on an annual basis to those EPs that continue to demonstrate meaningful use under rules of the CMS EHR Incentive Programs. We discuss attestation and compliance in more detail in chapter 11.

5

CHAPTER 6
Product Certification

Learn more about product certification.

Product certification is an important part of the meaningful use process. To stay on top of program updates and learn about changes associated with the product certification process, scan the QR code above or go to **certification.theMUguide.com.**

In this chapter, we explain what it means for technology to be certified for meaningful use. Regardless of whether you are a radiology IT vendor or group practice with in-house developed technology seeking certification, it is important for administrators and radiology EPs involved in meaningful use at your organization to understand what is required for product certification.

Using "certified" EHR technology

As part of the CMS EHR Incentive Programs, the U.S. Department of Health and Human Services (HHS) requires the use of "certified" technology by eligible providers and hospitals seeking funding under the American Recovery and Reinvestment Act (ARRA) of 2009.

The Office of the National Coordinator for Health IT (ONC) has established a temporary certification program to provide a way for organizations to become authorized by the ONC to test and certify EHR technology. The designation of ONC-Authorized Testing and Certification Bodies (ONC-ATCBs) identifies certification groups with approved certification programs that ensure EHRs are capable of meeting the 2011-2012 criteria for Stage 1 Meaningful Use.

Temporary EHR certification program

The temporary certification program was created to ensure that certified technology would be available for health care professionals looking to begin demonstrating meaningful use and collecting incentive payments starting in 2011. The temporary programs allow for the identification of authorized organizations that will test and certify EHR technology against the standards, implementation specifications, and certification criteria in place for the program. The current program will remain until a permanent certification program is established. The ONC will continue to work with the National Institute of Standards and Technology (NIST) in developing the permanent certification program no earlier than mid-2012.

Initial set of standards, implementation specifications, and certification criteria

ARRA legislation called for the ONC, in consultation with NIST, to develop a program for the voluntary certification of EHR technology. We have already discussed how the ONC established the temporary certification program, but it is NIST that is responsible for developing the functional and conformance testing requirements, test cases, and test tools in support of the health IT certification process.

Prior to the release of the Final Rule on July 13, 2010, NIST developed a series of draft procedures incorporating public feedback in the process. On July 13, 2010, NIST issued an initial set of standards, implementation specifications, and certification criteria to the ONC. The test procedures were approved and currently act as the basis for the temporary certification program used by ONC-ATCBs when certifying EHR technology. The following is a list of the all NIST Certification Criteria for Stage 1 Meaningful Use, including both EP and EH certification criteria (170.302 and 170.304 refer to EP criteria, while 170.306 refers to EH-specific criteria).

NIST CERTIFICATION CRITERIA

Number	NIST Certification Criteria and Description
45 CFR §170.302(a)	**Drug-drug, drug-allergy interaction checks.** (1) Notifications. Automatically and electronically generate in real-time at the point of care for drug-drug and drug-allergy contraindications based on medication list, medication allergy list, and computerized provider order entry (CPOE). (2) Adjustments. Provide certain users with the ability to adjust notifications provided for drug-drug and drug-allergy interaction checks.
45 CFR §170.302(b)	**Drug formulary checks.** Enable a user to electronically check if drugs are in a formulary or preferred drug list.
45 CFR §170.302(c)	**Maintain up-to-date problem list.** Enable a user to electronically record, modify, and retrieve a patient's problem list for longitudinal care in accordance with: (1) The standard specified in §170.207(a)(1); or (2) At a minimum, the version of the standard specified in §170.207(a)(2).
45 CFR §170.302(d)	**Maintain active medication list.** Enable a user to electronically record, modify, and retrieve a patient's active medication list as well as medication history for longitudinal care.
45 CFR §170.302(e)	**Maintain active medication allergy list.** Enable a user to electronically record, modify, and retrieve a patient's active medication allergy list as well as medication allergy history for longitudinal care.

Number	NIST Certification Criteria and Description
45 CFR §170.302(f)(1)	**Record and chart vital signs.** Enable a user to electronically record, modify, and retrieve a patient's vital signs including, at a minimum, the height, weight, and blood pressure.
45 CFR §170.302(f)(2)	**Calculate body mass index.** Automatically calculate and display body mass index (BMI) based on a patient's height and weight.
45 CFR §170.302(f)(3)	**Plot and display growth charts.** Plot and electronically display, upon request, growth charts for patients 2–20 years old.
45 CFR §170.302(g)	**Smoking status.** Enable a user to electronically record, modify, and retrieve the smoking status of a patient. Smoking status types must include: current everyday smoker; current some days smoker; former smoker; never smoker; smoker, current status unknown; unknown if ever smoked.
45 CFR §170.302(h)	**Incorporate laboratory test results.** (1) Receive results. Electronically receive clinical laboratory test results in a structured format and display such results in human readable format. (2) Display test report information. Electronically display all the information for a test report specified at 42 CFR 493.1291(c)(1) through (7). (3) Incorporate results. Electronically attribute, associate, or link a laboratory test result to a laboratory order or patient record.
45 CFR §170.302(i)	**Generate patient lists.** Enable a user to electronically select, sort, retrieve, and generate lists of patients according to, at a minimum, the data elements included in: (1) Problem list; (2) Medication list; (3) Demographics; and (4) Laboratory test results.
45 CFR §170.302(j)	**Medication reconciliation.** Enable a user to electronically compare two or more medication lists.
45 CFR §170.302(k)	**Submission to immunization registries.** Electronically record, modify, retrieve, and submit immunization information in accordance with: (1) the standard (and applicable implementation specifications) specified in §170.205(e)(1) or §170.205(e)(2); and (2) At a minimum, the version of the standard specified in §170.207(e).
45 CFR §170.302(l)	**Public health surveillance.** Electronically record, modify, retrieve, and submit syndrome-based public health surveillance information in accordance with the standard (and applicable implementation specifications) specified in §170.205(d)(1) or §170.205(d)(2).

Number	NIST Certification Criteria and Description
45 CFR §170.302(m)	**Patient-specific education resources.** Enable a user to electronically identify and provide patient-specific education resources according to, at a minimum, the data elements included in the patient's: problem list; medication list; and laboratory test results as well as provide such resources to the patient.
45 CFR §170.302(n)	**Automated measure calculation.** For each meaningful use objective with a percentage-based measure, electronically record the numerator and denominator and generate a report including the numerator, denominator, and resulting percentage associated with each applicable meaningful use measure.
45 CFR §170.302(o)	**Access control.** Assign a unique name and/or number for identifying and tracking user identity and establish controls that permit only authorized users to access electronic health information.
45 CFR §170.302(p)	**Emergency access.** Permit authorized users (who are authorized for emergency situations) to access electronic health information during an emergency.
45 CFR §170.302(q)	**Automatic log-off.** Terminate an electronic session after a predetermined time of inactivity.
45 CFR §170.302(r)	**Audit log.** (1) Record Actions. Record actions related to electronic health information in accordance with the standard specified in 170.210(b). (2) Generate audit log. Enable a user to generate an audit log for a specific time period and to sort entries in the audit log according to any of the elements specified in the standard at 170.210(b).
45 CFR §170.302(s)	**Integrity.** (1) Create a message digest in accordance with the standard specified in 170.210(c). (2) Verify in accordance with the standard specified in 170.210(c) upon receipt of electronically exchanged health information that such information has not been altered. (3) Detection. Detect the alteration of audit logs.
45 CFR §170.302(t)	**Authentication.** Verify that a person or entity seeking access to electronic health information is the one claimed and is authorized to access such information.

Number	NIST Certification Criteria and Description
45 CFR §170.302(u)	**General encryption.** Encrypt and decrypt electronic health information in accordance with the standard specified in §170.210(a)(1), unless the Secretary determines that the use of such algorithm would pose a significant security risk for certified EHR technology.
45 CFR §170.302(v)	**Encryption when exchanging electronic health information.** Encrypt and decrypt electronic health information when exchanged in accordance with the standard specified in §170.210(a)(2).
45 CFR §170.302(w)	**Accounting of disclosures (optional).** Record disclosures made for treatment, payment, and health care operations in accordance with the standards specified in §170.210(d).
45 CFR §170.304(a)	**Computerized provider order entry.** Enable a user to electronically record, store, retrieve, and modify, at a minimum, the following order types: (1) Medications; (2) Laboratory; and (3) Radiology/imaging.
45 CFR §170.304(b)	**Electronic prescribing.** Enable a user to electronically generate and transmit prescriptions and prescription-related information in accordance with: (1) The standard specified in §170.205(b)(1) or §170.205(b)(2); and (2) The standard specified in §170.207(d).
45 CFR §170.304(c)	**Record demographics.** Enable a user to electronically record, modify, and retrieve patient demographic data including preferred language, gender, race, ethnicity, and date of birth. Enable race and ethnicity to be recorded in accordance with the standard specified at §170.207(f).
45 CFR §170.304(d)	**Patient reminders.** Enable a user to electronically generate a patient reminder list for preventive or follow-up care according to patient preferences based on, at a minimum, the data elements included in: problem list; medication list; medication allergy list; demographics; and laboratory test results.
45 CFR §170.304(e)	**Clinical decision support.** (1) Implement rules. Implement automated, electronic clinical decision support rules (in addition to drug-drug and drug-allergy contraindication checking) based on the data elements included in: problem list; medication list; demographics; and laboratory test results. (2) Notifications. Automatically and electronically generate notifications and care suggestions based upon clinical decision support rules in real time.

Number	NIST Certification Criteria and Description
45 CFR §170.304(f)	**Electronic copy of health information.** Enable a user to create an electronic copy of a patient's clinical information, including, at a minimum, diagnostic test results, problem list, medication list, and medication allergy list in: (1) Human readable format; and (2) On electronic media or through some other electronic means in accordance with: (i) The standard (and applicable implementation specifications) specified in §170.205(a)(1) or §170.205(a)(2); and (ii) For the following data elements the applicable standard must be used: (A) Problems. The standard specified in §170.207(a)(1) or, at a minimum, the version of the standard specified in §170.207(a)(2); (B) Laboratory test results. At a minimum, the version of the standard specified in §170.207(c); and (C) Medications. The standard specified in §170.207(d).
45 CFR §170.304(g)	**Timely access.** Enable a user to provide patients with online access to their clinical information, including, at a minimum, lab test results, problem list, medication list, and medication allergy list.
45 CFR §170.304(h)	**Clinical summaries.** Enable a user to provide clinical summaries to patients for each office visit that include, at a minimum, diagnostic test results, problem list, medication list, and medication allergy list. If the clinical summary is provided electronically it must be: (1) Provided in human readable format; and (2) Provided on electronic media or through some other electronic means in accordance with: (i) The standard (and applicable implementation specifications) specified in §170.205(a)(1) or §170.205(a)(2); and (ii) For the following data elements the applicable standard must be used: (A) Problems. The standard specified in §170.207(a)(1) or, at a minimum, the version of the standard specified in §170.207(a)(2); (B) Laboratory test results. At a minimum, the version of the standard specified in §170.207(c); and (C) Medications. The standard specified in §170.207(d).

Number	NIST Certification Criteria and Description
45 CFR §170.304(i)	**Exchange clinical information and patient summary record.** (1) Electronically receive and display. Electronically receive and display a patient's summary record from other providers and organizations including, at a minimum, diagnostic test results, problem list, medication list, and medication allergy list in accordance with the standard (and applicable implementation specifications) specified in §170.205(a)(1) or §170.205(a)(2). Upon receipt of a patient summary record formatted in the alternative standard, display it in human readable format. (2) Electronically transmit. Enable a user to electronically transmit a patient summary record to other providers and organizations including, at a minimum, diagnostic test results, problem list, medication list, and medication allergy list in accordance with: (i) The standard (and applicable implementation specifications) specified in §170.205(a)(1) or §170.205(a)(2); and (ii) For the following data elements the applicable standard must be used: (A) Problems. The standard specified in §170.207(a)(1) or, at a minimum, the version of the standard specified in §170.207(a)(2); (B) Laboratory test results. At a minimum, the version of the standard specified in §170.207(c); and (C) Medications. The standard specified in §170.207(d).
45 CFR §170.304(j)	**Calculate and submit clinical quality measures.** (1) Calculate. (i) Electronically calculate all of the core clinical measures specified by CMS for eligible professionals. (ii) Electronically calculate, at a minimum, three clinical quality measures specified by CMS for eligible professionals, in addition to those clinical quality measures specified in paragraph (1)(i). (2) Submission. Enable a user to electronically submit calculated clinical quality measures in accordance with the standard and implementation specifications specified in §170.205(f).
45 CFR §170.306(a) (for EHs only)	**Computerized provider order entry.** Enable a user to electronically record, store, retrieve, and modify, at a minimum, the following order types: (1) Medications; (2) Laboratory; and (3) Radiology/Imaging.
45 CFR §170.306(b) (for EHs only)	**Record demographics.** Enable a user to electronically record, modify, and retrieve patient demographic data including preferred language, gender, race, ethnicity, date of birth, and date and preliminary cause of death in the event of mortality. Enable race and ethnicity to be recorded in accordance with the standard specified at §170.207(f).

Number	NIST Certification Criteria and Description
45 CFR §170.306(c) (for EHs only)	**Clinical decision support.** (1) Implement rules. Implement automated, electronic clinical decision support rules (in addition to drug-drug and drug-allergy contraindication checking) based on the data elements included in: problem list; medication list; demographics; and laboratory test results. (2) Notifications. Automatically and electronically generate and indicate in real-time, notifications and care suggestions based upon clinical decision support rules.
45 CFR §170.306(d)(1) (for EHs only)	**Electronic copy of health information.** (1) Enable a user to create an electronic copy of a patient's clinical information, including, at a minimum, diagnostic test results, problem list, medication list, medication allergy list, and procedures: (i) In human readable format; and (ii) On electronic media or through some other electronic means in accordance with: (A) The standard (and applicable implementation specifications) specified in §170.205(a)(1) or §170.205(a)(2); and (B) For the following data elements the applicable standard must be used: (1) Problems. The standard specified in §170.207(a)(1) or, at a minimum, the version of the standard specified in §170.207(a)(2); (2) Procedures. The standard specified in §170.207(b)(1) or §170.207(b)(2); (3) Laboratory test results. At a minimum, the version of the standard specified in §170.207(c); and (4) Medications. The standard specified in §170.207(d).
45 CFR §170.306(d)(2) (for EHs only)	**Electronic copy of health information (for discharge summaries).** (2) Enable a user to create an electronic copy of a patient's discharge summary in human readable format and on electronic media or through some other electronic means.
45 CFR §170.306(e) (for EHs only)	**Electronic copy of discharge instructions.** Enable a user to create an electronic copy of the discharge instructions for a patient, in human readable format, at the time of discharge on electronic media or through some other electronic means.

Number	NIST Certification Criteria and Description
45 CFR §170.306(f) (for EHs only)	**Exchange clinical information and patient summary record.** (1) Electronically receive and display. Electronically receive and display a patient's summary record from other providers and organizations including, at a minimum, diagnostic test results, problem list, medication list, medication allergy list, and procedures in accordance with the standard (and applicable implementation specifications) specified in §170.205(a)(1) or §170.205(a)(2). Upon receipt of a patient summary record formatted in the alternative standard, display it in human readable format. (2) Electronically transmit. Enable a user to electronically transmit a patient's summary record to other providers and organizations including, at a minimum, diagnostic results, problem list, medication list, medication allergy list, and procedures in accordance with: (i) The standard (and applicable implementation specifications) specified in §170.205(a)(1) or §170.205(a)(2); and (ii) For the following data elements the applicable standard must be used: (A) Problems. The standard specified in §170.207(a)(1) or, at a minimum, the version of the standard specified in §170.207(a)(2); (B) Procedures. The standard specified in §170.207(b)(1) or §170.207(b)(2); (C) Laboratory test results. At a minimum, the version of the standard specified in §170.207(c); and (D) Medications. The standard specified in §170.207(d).
45 CFR §170.306(g) (for EHs only)	**Reportable lab results.** Electronically record, modify, retrieve, and submit reportable clinical lab results in accordance with the standard (and applicable implementation specifications) specified in §170.205(c) and, at a minimum, the version of the standard specified in §170.207(c).
45 CFR §170.306(h) (for EHs only)	**Advance directives.** Enable a user to electronically record whether a patient has an advance directive.
45 CFR §170.306(i) (for EHs only)	**Calculate and submit clinical quality measures.** (1) Calculate. Electronically calculate all of the clinical quality measures specified by CMS for eligible hospitals and critical access hospitals. (2) Submission. Enable a user to electronically submit calculated clinical quality measures in accordance with the standard and implementation specifications specified in §170.205(f).

Source: National Institute of Standards and Technology.

Stay Up-to-Date: NIST updates will be conducted through a standard maintenance process and updated test procedures will be released every six months. For an up-to-date list of NIST criteria and updated test procedures, scan the QR code at the beginning of this chapter or go to **certification.theMUguide.com.**

Note that for radiology and all other medical specialties, test procedures will not be modified to be domain or specialty specific. The certification program addresses how an ONC-ATCB may consider any unique aspects of domain and specialty systems. For more information about the structure of the test procedures for evaluating conformance of complete and modular EHR technology against the certification criteria defined in 45 CFR 170 Subpart C of the Final Rule, visit the NIST website. You can also find referenced standards and implementation specifications (45 CFR 170.205, 170.207, and 170.210) that are associated with specific certification criteria on the NIST website.

Meaningful Use Objectives vs. NIST Certification Criteria

The following table maps the meaningful use objectives against the NIST Certification Criteria required for EHR product certification. This list is relevant for EPs participating in the Medicare EHR Incentive Program.

Meaningful Use Objectives	NIST Certification Criteria
42 CFR §495.6(d)(1): Use CPOE for medication order directly entered by any licensed health care professional who can enter orders into the medical record per state, local, and professional guidelines	**45 CFR §170.304(a):** Computerized provider order entry
42 CFR §495.6(d)(2): Implement drug-drug and drug-allergy interaction checks	**45 CFR §170.302(a):** Drug-drug, drug-allergy interaction checks
42 CFR §495.6(d)(3): Maintain an up-to-date problem list of current and active diagnoses	**45 CFR §170.302(c):** Maintain up-to-date problem list
42 CFR §495.6(d)(4): Generate and transmit permissible prescriptions electronically (eRx)	**45 CFR §170.304(b):** Electronic prescribing
42 CFR §495.6(d)(5): Maintain active medication list	**45 CFR §170.302(d):** Maintain active medication list
42 CFR §495.6(d)(6): Maintain active medication allergy list	**45 CFR §170.302(e):** Maintain active medication allergy list

Meaningful Use Objectives	NIST Certification Criteria
42 CFR §495.6(d)(7): Record demographics (preferred language, gender, race, ethnicity, date of birth)	**45 CFR §170.304(c):** Record demographics
42 CFR §495.6(d)(8): Record and chart changes in vital signs (height, weight, blood pressure, calculate and display BMI, plot and display growth charts for children 2–20 years including BMI)	**45 CFR §170.302(f):** Record and chart vital signs
42 CFR §495.6(d)(9): Record smoking status for patients 13 years old or older	**45 CFR §170.302(g):** Smoking status
42 CFR §495.6(d)(10): Report ambulatory clinical quality measures to CMS	**45 CFR §170.304(j):** Calculate and submit clinical quality measures
42 CFR §495.6(d)(11): Implement one clinical decision support rule relevant to specialty or high clinical priority along with the ability to track compliance with that rule	**45 CFR §170.304(e):** Clinical decision support
42 CFR §495.6(d)(12): Provide patients with an electronic copy of their health information (including diagnostic test results, problem list, medication list, medication allergies) upon request	**45 CFR §170.304(f):** Electronic copy of health information
42 CFR §495.6(d)(13): Provide clinical summaries for patients for each office visit	**45 CFR §170.304(h):** Clinical summaries
42 CFR §495.6(d)(14): Capability to exchange key clinical information (for example, problem list, medication list, medication allergies, diagnostic test results) among providers of care and patient-authorized entities electronically	**45 CFR §170.304(i):** Exchange clinical information and patient summary record
42 CFR §495.6(d)(15): Protect electronic health information created or maintained by the certified EHR technology through the implementation of appropriate technical capabilities	**45 CFR §170.302(o):** Access control **45 CFR §170.302(p):** Emergency access **45 CFR §170.302(q):** Automatic log-off **45 CFR §170.302(r):** Audit log **45 CFR §170.302(s):** Integrity **45 CFR §170.302(t):** Authentication **45 CFR §170.302(u):** General encryption **45 CFR §170.302(v):** Encryption when exchanging electronic health information **45 CFR §170.302(w - optional):** Accounting of disclosures

Meaningful Use Objectives	NIST Certification Criteria
42 CFR §495.6(e)(1): Implement drug-formulary checks	**45 CFR §170.302(b):** Drug-formulary checks
42 CFR §495.6(e)(2): Incorporate clinical lab test results into EHR as structured data	**45 CFR §170.302(h):** Incorporate laboratory test results
42 CFR §495.6(e)(3): Generate lists of patients by specific conditions to use for quality improvement, reduction of disparities, research, or outreach	**45 CFR §170.302(i):** Generate patient lists
42 CFR §495.6(e)(4): Send reminders to patients per patient preference for preventive/follow-up care	**45 CFR §170.304(d):** Patient reminders
42 CFR §495.6(e)(5): Provide patients with timely electronic access to their health information (including lab results, problem list, medication list, medication allergies) within four business days of the information being available to the EP	**45 CFR §170.304(g):** Timely access
42 CFR §495.6(e)(6): Use certified EHR technology to identify patient-specific education resources and provide those resources to the patient if appropriate	**45 CFR §170.302(m):** Patient-specific education resources
42 CFR §495.6(e)(7): The EP who receives a patient from another setting of acre or provider of care or believes an en-counter is relevant should perform medication reconciliation	**45 CFR §170.302(j):** Medication reconciliation
42 CFR §495.6(e)(8): The EP who transitions their patient to another setting of care or provider of care or refers their patient to another provider of care should provide summary of care record for each transition of care or referral	**45 CFR §170.304(i):** Exchange clinical information and patient summary record
42 CFR §495.6(e)(9): Capability to submit electronic data to immunization registries or immunization information systems and actual submission according to applicable law and practice	**45 CFR §170.302(k):** Submission to immunization registries
42 CFR §495.6(e)(10): Capability to submit electronic syndromic surveillance data to public health agencies and actual submission according to applicable law and practice	**45 CFR §170.302(l):** Public health surveillance
N/A	**45 CFR §170.302(n):** Automated measure calculation

ONC-Authorized Testing and Certification Bodies (ONC-ATCBs)

As discussed earlier, the Office of the National Coordinator for Health IT (ONC) Authorized Testing and Certification Bodies (ATCBs) identifies certification groups with approved certification programs that ensure EHRs are capable of meeting the 2011-2012 criteria for Stage 1 Meaningful Use. The use of "certified" technology is required by the U.S. Department of Health and Human Services (HHS) for eligible providers and hospitals seeking funding under the American Recovery and Reinvestment Act (ARRA) of 2009.

At the time of this writing, there are five ONC-ATCB certification groups that are authorized to certify Complete EHR technology and one group authorized to certify ePrescribing, Privacy, and Security EHR modules only. Each certification body offers complete and modular certification as well as onsite, offsite, and remote certification programs.

The organizations listed below have been authorized to perform Complete EHR and/or EHR Module testing and certification. These ONC-ATCBs are required to test and certify EHRs to the applicable certification criteria adopted by the Secretary under subpart C of Part 170 Part II and Part III as stipulated in the Standards and Certification Criteria Final Rule. Certification by an ATCB will signify to eligible professionals, hospitals, and critical access hospitals that EHR technology has the capabilities necessary to support their efforts to meet the goals and objectives of meaningful use.

- **Certification Commission for Health Information Technology (CCHIT®):** CCHIT has been recognized by the Office of the National Coordinator for Health Information Technology (ONC) and U.S. Department of Health and Human Services (HHS) as an Authorized Testing and Certification Body (ATCB) for the purposes of certifying that EHRs are capable of meeting the government developed criteria to support meaningful use and qualify eligible providers and hospitals for funding under the American Recovery and Reinvestment Act (ARRA). For more information, go to **cchit.theMUguide.com.**

- **Drummond Group®:** The Drummond Group provides highly effective and efficient electronic health record (EHR) testing to healthcare information technology vendors. As an Office of the National Coordinator Authorized Testing and Certification Body (ONC-ATCB), they work closely with healthcare information technology vendors and hospitals to certify their EHR software for use by health care providers looking to qualify for incentive funds under the American Recovery and Reinvestment Act (ARRA). All eligible professionals, eligible hospitals, and critical access hospitals must adopt and successfully demonstrate meaningful use of certified EHR technology to qualify for these incentive monies. For more information, go to **drummond.theMUguide.com.**

- **InfoGard Laboratories:** InfoGard performs both Complete EHR and EHR Module test and certification as an ONC-ATCB. They provide onsite testing at the vendor facility, remote testing, or testing at their facility to support the needs and success of their customers. They have a test plan and test preparedness documentation to ensure the EHR vendor is well prepared for testing. They also provide a test preparedness service for those EHR vendors who need assistance in understanding the criteria and the test requirements, determining if their EHR product is compliant, and in fully preparing for the testing. For more information, go to **infogard.theMUguide.com.**

- **ICSA Labs:** ICSA Labs is an independent division of Verizon Business, a unit of Verizon Communications which offers vendor-neutral testing and certification of security products and solutions for hundreds of the world's top security vendors. No stranger to the medical industry, they certify MDex, the medical data exchange for dictated medical information. Together with the Medical Transcription Industry Association (MTIA) they have created the Medical Transcription Service Consortium (MTSC) to promote this secure exchange. For more information, go to **icsalabs.theMUguide.com.**

- **SLI Global Solutions:** Based in Denver with global offices, SLI offers technology risk and investment management. They are an ONC-ATCB and their Corporate Quality System (CQS) has been audited to and certified against ISO 9001:2008 standards of quality performance. SLI is also a certified lab under the National Voluntary Laboratory Accreditation Program (NVLAP) of the National Institute of Standards and Technology (NIST). This, coupled with their extensive knowledge of healthcare IT systems, qualifies SLI to provide all of your certification needs. For more information, go to **sliglobal.theMUguide.com.**

- **Surescripts (ePrescribing, Privacy, and Security modules only):** Surescripts operates the nation's largest e-prescription network and supports a rapidly expanding ecosystem of health care organizations nationwide. Surescripts was founded on the principles of neutrality, transparency, interoperability, efficiency, collaboration, and quality. For more information, go to **surescripts.theMUguide.com.**

Stay Up-to-Date: For the latest list of authorized testing bodies, scan the QR code at the beginning of this chapter or go to **certification.theMUguide.com.**

Below is a quick comparison of ONC-ATCBs as of late 2011. Prices vary from one provider to another and some certification groups charge for additional services such as onsite testing and certification retesting, while others do not.

COMPARISON OF ONC-ATCBs

ONC-ATCB	Authorization	Testing Model	Complete Ambulatory EHR Certification Cost	Modular Ambulatory EHR Certification Cost
Certification Commission for Health Information Technology (CCHIT)	Complete and Modular EHR	Onsite and Remote	$34,300	$7,000 base fee plus $650–2,000 per certification criteria based on complexity
Drummond Group	Complete and Modular EHR	Onsite and Remote	$19,500	$6,000–16,000 based on number of modules
InfoGard Laboratories	Complete and Modular EHR	Onsite and Remote	$19,900	$5,000 (includes eight security and privacy modules plus one additional module)
ICSA Labs	Complete and Modular EHR	Onsite and Remote	N/A	N/A
SLI Global Solutions	Complete and Modular EHR	Remote	$20,000	$6,000–15,000 based on number of modules
Surescripts	Modular EHR (ePrescribing, Privacy, and Security modules only)	Onsite and Remote	N/A	Free

Source: radiologyMU.org.

Stay Up-to-Date: The list of current and active ONC-ATCBs, and their cost averages, has the potential to change. For an up-to-date list of all current ONC-ATCBs, certification details, and estimated costs, scan the QR code at the beginning of this chapter or go to **certification.theMUguide.com.**

Complete EHR certification vs. Modular EHR certification

Every vendor (and any health care provider looking to certify technology) needs to have their technology certified by an ONC-ATCB as Complete or Modular EHR technology. Complete EHR certification means the technology has been certified to meet all 33 mandatory certification criteria as identified in the Standards and Certification Criteria Final Rule (45 CFR Part 170 Part III). Modular EHR certification means the technology has been certified for at least one of the certification criteria, in addition to the privacy and security criteria, as defined in the Standards and Certification Criteria Final Rule. The following privacy and security criteria, with the exception of 45 CFR §170.302(w), which is optional, are required for all modular certified EHRs:

- **45 CFR §170.302(o):** Access control.

- **45 CFR §170.302(p):** Emergency access.

- **45 CFR §170.302(q):** Automatic log-off.

- **45 CFR §170.302(r):** Audit log.

- **45 CFR §170.302(s):** Integrity.

- **45 CFR §170.302(t):** Authentication.

- **45 CFR §170.302(u):** General encryption.

- **45 CFR §170.302(v):** Encryption when exchanging electronic health information.

- **45 CFR §170.302(w - optional):** Accounting of disclosures.

Any technology, including radiology IT software such as your RIS, PACS, Reporting, or other technology, can be either certified as a Complete EHR or a module. As such, your imaging practice can combine modularly certified products to achieve meaningful use. If you choose to combine EHR modules, you need to be certain that they cover all of your meaningful use requirements. Also, the ONC regulations currently state you need to "possess" all certification criteria, even if you don't use them for your meaningful use measures. This is an important requirement that could change in future regulations.

ONC FAQ: 9-10-017-2

Question: I am an eligible health care provider seeking to achieve "meaningful use of Certified EHR Technology" under the Medicare and Medicaid EHR Incentive Programs. I understand that under the Medicare and Medicaid EHR Incentive Programs ("meaningful use") Final Rule, I am permitted to defer up to 5 meaningful use "menu set" objectives and associated measures for a given EHR reporting period. Do I need to possess EHR technology that has/have been tested and certified: A) to all of the applicable certification criteria adopted in ONC's Standards and Certification Criteria Final Rule; or B) only to those certification criteria that correlate with the Stage 1 core set objectives and associated measures and menu set objectives and associated measures I select to report on to CMS?

Answer: "A - to all of the applicable certification criteria adopted in ONC's Standards and Certification Criteria Final Rule." Eligibility to receive a Medicare or Medicaid EHR Incentive Payment consists of two related, but distinct steps—the possession of Certified EHR Technology and subsequently demonstrating its meaningful use. In order to be able to attest to CMS or States at the end of your EHR reporting period that you possess EHR technology that meets the regulatory definition of Certified EHR Technology adopted by HHS (45 CFR 170.102 and 42 CFR 495.4), the EHR technology in your possession must have been tested and certified to all applicable certification criteria adopted for the setting (ambulatory or inpatient) for which it was designed (see also CMS FAQ 10162). Please see the discussion below for more on the meaning of "applicable certification criteria" as well as what is required for the EHR technology in your possession to meet the definition of Certified EHR Technology.

To view the "possess" FAQ online, scan the QR code at the beginning of this chapter or go to **certification.theMUguide.com**.

Product certification process

As part of the Final Rule, the ONC has issued standard guidelines for which all ONC-ATCBs must adhere. While the exact step-by-step certification process varies slightly from one ONC-ATCB to another, it typically includes five primary phases—material review, application, pretesting, testing, and certification. Although all ONC-ATCBs are required to adhere to NIST testing guidelines, the exact manner in which testing procedures and scripts are presented to an organization seeking EHR certification varies.

In general, the process begins with a review of program materials, product eligibility requirements, and initial test script review. Once completed, the application phase typically follows. This is simply the formal process of applying for product certification with your ONC-ATCB of choice.

Next, organizations seeking certification of their EHR products will complete a pretesting phase. During this phase, a questionnaire will typically be required in order to create a custom test plan and guidance material will often be supplied. This phase also frequently involves a walk-through of testing and identification of potential non-compliance prior to the official testing phase.

Once pretesting has been successfully completed, the testing phase is conducted. Many ONC-ATCBs offer both onsite (at their facility or the EHR vendor's facility) and remote testing (conducted via remote desktop software). During this phase, if a product fails to comply with any testing requirements, the product is subject to retesting at the vendors expense, if applicable.

Finally, after all requirements are successfully met, certification is granted for the product and software version that was tested. Once certified, the ONC-ATCB will notify the ONC and details will be submitted to the ONC Certified HIT Product List (CHPL). Lastly, the certified product vendor will receive a certificate that identifies product certification details as well as a design mark from the ONC-ATCB for marketing purposes.

Certifying your own imaging technology

If your imaging practice has developed EHR technology and your group plans to use the technology to demonstrate meaningful use, you will need to approach product certification in the same manner as a healthcare IT vendor. Studying the regulations and analyzing your EHR technology against the 33 Certification Criteria is imperative to product certification success. It is also important to note that the entire process, from initial planning through final certification, can take anywhere from six to eighteen months depending on the degree of product modifications that are required to meet all required certification criteria.

6

CHAPTER 7
Meaningful Use for Radiologists

Find out more about how meaningful use impacts radiologists.

Meaningful use is evolving and its impact on radiology EPs is in a constant state of flux. For the latest information about how the incentive programs affect radiologists, scan the QR code above or go to **radiologists.theMUguide.com.**

In this chapter, we build on what we've already learned and look closer at how it affects the radiology community. This includes a discussion of multi-site imaging practice environments, specific financial implications of the program, clarifications and guidance, and challenges for radiology professionals.

Meaningful use for radiologists

Stage 1 of the CMS EHR Incentive Programs clearly focuses on the primary care physician and takes a one-size-fits-all view with respect to all eligible professionals. It's this approach, coupled with the dissemination of old information released prior to the Final Rule in July 2010, that has led to considerable confusion amongst radiologists, chief information officers, radiology IT directors/managers, and diagnostic imaging IT vendors.

Despite the misunderstanding that meaningful use does not apply to diagnostic imaging professionals, it's well known that the majority of U.S.-based radiologists are eligible for the Medicare version of the CMS EHR Incentive Programs and the potential financial upside. What's more, eligible radiologists are also on the hook for nonparticipation penalties beginning in 2015.

While there are considerable challenges associated with this legislation that is not tailored for the medical imaging specialist, there is help on the horizon. In the radiology domain, IT vendors—including RIS, PACS, Reporting, Decision Support, Image Sharing, Patient Portal, and Business Analytics providers—are actively applying for certification of their technology and solutions. In fact, a number of radiology-specific certified EHR technologies already exist today. However, the exact number of criteria that each product will be certified for will vary from vendor to vendor. This variability translates into radiologists and practice managers needing to determine which combination of certified products and functionality they will use to achieve meaningful use in the cases where a complete certified solution does not exist.

Advent of the "imaging EMR"

The notion of an EMR for radiologists, or an imaging EMR, is creating a new breed of information systems for diagnostic imaging professionals. These enhanced systems are capable of doing more than a traditional radiology IT system in terms of recording and measuring data for expanding IT initiatives. To achieve meaningful use with a traditional radiology IT system, most technology providers will need to add components to their offering that are typically present in a traditional EMR system. An increasing number of healthcare IT providers are embedding this required EMR functionality into the RIS and other radiology IT systems to satisfy the requirements of meaningful use. As more imaging practices make progress with Stage 1 Meaningful Use, they will seek technology that supports their incentive program strategies and drive the development and adoption of imaging EMRs.

Financial impact on the imaging community and your organization

The overall impact of the CMS EHR Incentive Programs on the medical imaging community is estimated at well over $1 billion. While the incentive opportunities are substantial, the potential for ongoing penalties cannot be overlooked. Incentives are the clear upside today, but the potential for payment reductions after 2015 will ultimately become a more significant motivator over time.

These initiatives have the potential to add measurable value to your imaging practice. Using a seven-year cost analysis—including technology costs, incentive opportunities, and potential penalties—individual imaging practices stand to gain anywhere from $150,000 (small imaging practice) all the way up to more than $8 million (large academic medical practice) over the full term of the incentive payment period. This is of course based on the number of EPs in your practice and on an assumption that your group is able to begin demonstrating meaningful use by 2012 to reap full incentive opportunities and continues doing so for the remainder of the incentive payment period.

In chapter 8, we discuss methods for determining the financial impact of this incentive program using your own imaging practice data.

Providing imaging services in multiple locations

If you have radiology EPs that provide imaging services in more than one practice or location, more than half of their patient encounters must come from locations which possess certified EHR technology. Since meaningful use requirements are measured for locations that possess certified EHR technology, any patient encounters that take place at locations without certified EHR technology are not counted toward radiology EP measure calculations. Furthermore, if an EP sees patients in both inpatient and outpatient settings possessing certified EHR technology, the EP should base their program calculations on patients in the outpatient setting only.

"Seen by the EP" clarification and guidance for radiologists

On June 6, 2011, CMS published guidance that could enhance the ability of radiologists to comply with meaningful use program requirements. The verbiage "seen by the EP" originally implied that any service rendered by the EP, in this case the radiologist, should be included in final meaningful use measure calculations. The implication of the guidance released by CMS in June 2011 indicates that a diagnostic radiologist could conceivably choose to limit their "seen" patients to physical visits, omitting teleradiology and similar services, for meaningful use measures that include "seen by the EP" verbiage. While there is flexibility in the current language, CMS does require that the EP have a consistent policy on when to include or omit these patients from their calculations. In addition, a secondary FAQ was published the same day indicating that when a patient is seen by the EP's clinical staff and not the EP themselves, the EP can elect to include or not include those patients in their meaningful use calculations as long as the decision applies universally to all patients across the required measures.

CMS FAQ: How does an EP determine whether a patient has been "seen by the EP"...*Published 06/06/2011 09:58 AM | Answer ID 10664*

Question: For the Medicare and Medicaid EHR Incentive Programs, how does an eligible professional (EP) determine whether a patient has been "seen by the EP" in cases where the service rendered does not result in an actual interaction between the patient and the EP, but minimal consultative services such as just reading an EKG? Is a patient seen via telemedicine included in the denominator for measures that include patients "seen by the EP?"

Answer: All cases where the EP and the patient have an actual physical encounter with the patient in which they render any service to the patient should be included in the denominator as "seen by the EP." A patient seen through telemedicine would also count as a patient "seen by the EP." However, in cases where the EP and the patient do not have an actual physical or telemedicine encounter, but the EP renders a minimal consultative service for the patient (like reading an EKG), the EP may choose whether to include the patient in the denominator as "seen by the EP" provided the choice is consistent for the entire EHR reporting period and for all relevant meaningful use measures. For example, a cardiologist may choose to exclude patients for whom they provide a one-time reading of an EKG sent to them from another provider, but include more involved consultative services as long as the policy is consistent for the entire EHR reporting period and for all meaningful use measures that include patients "seen by the EP." EPs who never have a physical or telemedicine interaction with patients must adopt a policy that classifies as least some of the services they render for patients as "seen by the EP" and this policy must be consistent for the entire EHR reporting period and across meaningful use measures that involve patients "seen by the EP"— otherwise, these EPs would not be able to satisfy meaningful use, as they would have denominators of zero for some measures.

CMS FAQ: When a patient is only seen by a member of the EP's clinical staff during the EHR reporting period...*Published 06/06/2011 10:10 AM | Answer ID 10665*

Question: For the Medicare and Medicaid EHR Incentive Programs, when a patient is only seen by a member of the eligible professional's (EP's) clinical staff during the EHR reporting period and not by the EP themselves, do those patients count in the EP's denominator?

Answer: The EP can include or not include those patients in their denominator at their discretion as long as the decision applies universally to all patients for the entire EHR reporting period and the EP is consistent across meaningful use measures. In cases where a member of the EP's clinical staff is eligible for the Medicaid EHR Incentive Program in their own right (NPs and certain physician assistants (PAs)), patients seen by NPs or PAs under the EP's supervision can be counted by both the NP or PA and the supervising EP as long as the policy is consistent for the entire EHR reporting period.

To view the "seen by the EP" FAQs online, scan the QR code at the beginning of this chapter or go to **radiologists.theMUguide.com.**

"Seen by the EP" meaningful use measures

The following is a list of the nine core and menu set measures that contain "seen by the EP" terminology. Based on the guidance discussed above, these measures allow EPs to limit their "seen" patients to physical visits only.

- **42 CFR §495.6(d)(1):** More than 30% of unique patients with at least one medication in their medication list seen by the EP have at least one medication order entered using CPOE.

- **42 CFR §495.6(d)(3):** More than 80% of all unique patients seen by the EP have at least one entry or an indication that no problems are known for the patient recorded as structured data.

- **42 CFR §495.6(d)(5):** More than 80% of all unique patients seen by the EP have at least one entry (or an indication that the patient is not currently prescribed any medication) recorded as structured data.

- **42 CFR §495.6(d)(6):** More than 80% of all unique patients seen by the EP have at least one entry (or an indication that the patient has no known medication allergies) recorded as structured data.

- **42 CFR §495.6(d)(7):** More than 50% of all unique patients seen by the EP have demographics recorded as structured data.

- **42 CFR §495.6(d)(8):** More than 50% of all unique patients age 2 and over seen by the EP; height, weight and blood pressure are recorded as structured data.

- **42 CFR §495.6(d)(9):** More than 50% of all unique patients 13 years old or older seen by the EP have smoking status recorded as structured data.

- **42 CFR §495.6(e)(5):** More than 10% of all unique patients seen by the EP are provided timely (available to the patient within four business days of being updated in the certified EHR technology) electronic access to their health information subject to the EP's discretion to withhold certain information.

- **42 CFR §495.6(e)(6):** More than 10% of all unique patients seen by the EP during the EHR reporting period are provided patient-specific education resources.

As the program evolves, new statements containing clarification and guidance are likely to be published. For updates pertaining to this material, go to **radiologists.theMUguide.com.**

Challenges for radiology professionals

Even though recent clarifications assist radiologists in achieving meaningful use, this government program still presents a number of challenges for medical specialists like radiologists. However, careful planning and a focused approach will ensure your imaging practice's success with meaningful use. The following challenges exist for radiologists with respect to the CMS EHR Incentive Programs.

- Most radiologists are eligible as EPs for both incentives and penalties.

- Meaningful use was designed as a one-size-fits-all program.

- It is not necessarily clinically relevant technology for most radiologists.

- Radiology EPs may not have purchasing influence over their technology.

- Hospitals may purchase an inpatient EHR without an ambulatory EHR.

- Many radiology IT software solutions will only achieve modular certification.

- There is no flexibility in the 33 Certification Criteria requirements.

- Radiologists may need to "possess" additional certified EHR technology in order to comply with program requirements.

Despite these challenges, there is hope. More and more imaging professionals and technology providers are taking an interest in meaningful use every day. As a result, certified radiology solutions are being developed and experiences shared, leading to a more collaborative advance toward success. In the next part of this guide, we review a 10-step approach to tackling the obstacles and hurdles of meaningful use for radiologists.

Part II:

BUILDING YOUR STRATEGY: 10 STEPS TO ACHIEVING MEANINGFUL USE FOR RADIOLOGISTS

In Part II, we outline a proven 10-step strategy for radiology EPs to follow as they approach meaningful use—preparing, developing, executing, and sustaining a strategy for success. First, we start with preparation, including a review of meaningful use fundamentals, eligibility requirements, and the financial impact of this government program, as well as take an in-depth look at exclusion opportunities for typical radiology practice settings and work types. After that, we move on to developing your strategy through practice stakeholder meetings and discussions with radiology IT vendors. Next, we focus on execution of your strategy through technical and operational planning as well as acquiring and implementing new certified technology, if needed. Finally, we consider ways to sustain meaningful use including program registration, compliance-monitoring using dashboards and scorecards, and attesting with CMS.

CHAPTER 8
Preparing for Meaningful Use

STEP 1:
Understanding the fundamentals
of meaningful use

STEP 2:
Determining your eligibility and financial
impact of the program

STEP 3:
Determining your meaningful use
measure requirements

Prepare yourself for meaningful use.

To further educate yourself on program fundamentals, access updated resource links,
download helpful worksheets, and run an analysis on your imaging practice, scan the QR
code above or go to **prepare.theMUguide.com.**

In this first chapter of the 10-step approach to achieving meaningful use, we discuss recommendations for understanding program fundamentals, determining your eligibility, and assessing the financial impact. We also help you determine your radiology EP meaningful use measure requirements.

STEP 1:
Understanding the fundamentals of meaningful use

Meaningful use success begins with understanding the fundamentals. Whether that means visiting the government program website, going to lectures, reading articles, listening to podcasts, attending tradeshows, or reading the nearly one thousand pages of regulations, it is imperative that you understand the fundamentals of the CMS EHR Incentive Programs and what they mean to your diagnostic imaging practice. In addition to familiarizing yourself with Part I of this guide, we recommend you use the following resources to better understand the fundamentals of meaningful use.

Radiology-specific online resources

While there are many resources available online with information about the CMS EHR Incentive Programs, there are a few key resources focused specifically on education and implications of these government programs for the radiology community.

- **radiologyMU.org:** This website provides eligible professionals (EPs) in the diagnostic imaging community with objective information about meaningful use as it relates to the field of medical imaging. This valuable resource offers a free online practice analyzer, community collaboration tools, and a mobile companion app for iOS devices (two versions; iPhone and iPad). Go to **radiologyMU.org.**

- **ACR MU Resource Center:** This page on the American College of Radiology website is a collection of resources and documents related to the Centers for Medicare and Medicaid Services EHR Incentive Programs. Go to **acr.theMUguide.com.**

Federal resources

These federal resources provide a wealth of information about meaningful use legislation, regulations, and program requirements.

- **CMS Medicare and Medicaid Electronic Heath Records (EHR) Incentive Programs Website:** The official website for the CMS EHR Incentive Programs with information and program details, registration links, attestation links, FAQs, and more. Go to **cms.theMUguide.com.**

- **The Office of the National Coordinator (ONC) for Health Information Technology:** The official website for the ONC. Go to **onc.theMUguide.com.**

- **Medicare and Medicaid Programs Electronic Health Record Incentive Program Final Rule:** This Final Rule implements the provisions of the American Recovery and Reinvestment Act (ARRA) of 2009 (Pub. L. 111-5) that provide incentive payments to eligible professionals (EPs), eligible hospitals (EHs), and critical access hospitals (CAHs) participating in Medicare and Medicaid programs that adopt and successfully demonstrate meaningful use of certified electronic health record (EHR) technology. This document specifies the initial criteria EPs, EHs, and CAHs must meet in order to qualify for an incentive payment; calculation of the incentive payment amounts; payment adjustments under Medicare for covered professional services and inpatient hospital services provided by EPs, EHs, and CAHs failing to demonstrate meaningful use of certified EHR technology; and other program participation requirements. Go to **cmsfinalrule.theMUguide.com.**

- **Comparison of Meaningful Use Objectives between the Proposed Rule and the Final Rule:** This brief document outlines the changes from the Proposed Rule to the Final Rule issued by CMS. Go to **comparison.theMUguide.com.**

- **Health Information Technology Initial Set of Standards, Implementation Specifications, and Certification Criteria for Electronic Health Record Technology Final Rule:** This document fully outlines the initial set of standards, implementation specifications, and certification criteria to ensure alignment with final Stage 1 Meaningful Use objectives and measures. Go to **oncfinalrule.theMUguide.com.**

- **Establishment of the Temporary Certification Program for Health Information Technology Final Rule:** This document is the Final Rule that establishes a temporary certification program for the purpose of certifying health information technology (HIT). Go to **tempcert.theMUguide.com.**

- **Establishment of the Permanent Certification Program for Health Information Technology:** This document is the Final Rule that establishes a permanent certification program for the purpose of certifying health information technology (HIT). Go to **permcert.theMUguide.com.**

- **Certified HIT Product List (CHPL):** This official program website provides the authoritative, comprehensive listing of Complete EHRs and EHR Modules that have been tested and certified under the Temporary Certification Program maintained by the Office of the National Coordinator for Health IT (ONC). Each Complete EHR and EHR Module listed on this website has been certified by an ONC-Authorized Testing and Certification Body (ONC-ATCB) and reported to ONC. Only the product versions that are included on the CHPL are certified under the ONC Temporary Certification Program. Go to **chpl.theMUguide.com.**

Program fact sheets

The official program fact sheets found on these government websites offer concise overviews and detailed information about the incentive programs.

- **Electronic Health Records at a Glance:** This fact sheet provides a concise overview of EHRs and answers such questions as why EHRs are held to meaningful use requirements, and provides a look ahead with timetables and an outline of the incentive program. Go to **ataglance.theMUguide.com.**

- **CMS and ONC Final Regulations Define Meaningful Use and Set Standards for Electronic Health Record Incentive Program:** This fact sheet discusses the Final CMS Rule, the Final ONC Rule, timetable for implementation, the meaningful use model, the approach to supporting EHR adoption, key provisions of the Final Rule, and insight into the development of the rules. Go to **definetheprogram.theMUguide.com.**

- **CMS Finalized Definition of Meaningful Use of Certified Electronic Health Records (EHR) Technology:** This fact sheet defines meaningful use policy goals, reviews the development of Stage 1 criteria, and discusses policy goals beyond Stage 1 Meaningful Use. Go to **definecertified.theMUguide.com.**

MU-related blogs and social media

There are a few official government blogs as well as social media resources, such as Twitter, that offer valuable information and updates about meaningful use.

- **Health IT Buzz Blog:** This blog is a service of the ONC and was created to answer questions and create a conversation about the challenges and successes health care providers and organizations are experiencing as they transition to Electronic Health Records. Go to **hitblog.theMUguide.com.**

- **Radiology and HIT Blog:** This blog is maintained by Michael Peters, Director of Legislative and Regulatory Affairs for the American College of Radiology (ACR), and discusses radiology and health IT policy news from the ACR Government Relations Team. Go to **radiologyblog.theMUguide.com.**

- **Federal Advisory Committee Blog:** Go to **facblog.theMUguide.com.**

- **Twitter:** Social media outlets such as Twitter are a fantastic resource for up-to-the-minute news, announcements, and updates related to meaningful use. To find MU-related content, we recommend searching with the following hashtags: **#MEANINGFULUSE #MU #HITECH #EHR #EMR #CMS #ONC.**

Step 2:
Determining your eligibility and financial impact

In chapter 7, we discussed how the Continuing Extension Act of 2010 shifted POS 22, and as a result, shifted the meaningful use eligibility status for most radiologists practicing in the United States. Even so, it is recommended that you review your own practice setting and group billing history to determine your eligibility for the incentive program and conduct a meaningful use analysis using your group's practice and individual EP data.

Preparing an analysis before developing your strategy not only helps you to better understand the impact of the Medicare EHR Incentive Program on your practice, but also provides a baseline for internal and external meaningful use discussions and planning. Fortunately, there are tools available online to assist with this process. In order to complete your online analysis, you must answer the following questions as well as questions outlined in the next step. Note that a worksheet with all required questions for both Step 2 and Step 3 is available for download from the online companion website. Eligibility and financial impact questions include:

- How many radiologists practice in your imaging group?

- What is your total CMS revenue for radiology services?

- Are you part of a multi-specialty practice?

- Does your practice plan to enroll and participate in the CMS EHR Incentive Programs?

- When do you plan to begin meaningful use of certified technology (Already enrolled, 10/3/2012, 10/3/2013, 10/3/2014, not until after 2015)?

- What percentage of your CMS volume is Inpatient Hospital (POS21)?

- What percentage of your CMS volume is Emergency Room (POS23)?

- Does your group practice in a Health Professional Shortage Area (HPSA)?

- Who is the supplier of your EHR/EMR(s)?

- Who is the supplier of your RIS(s)?

- Who is the supplier of your PACS(s)?

- Who is the supplier of your Radiology Reporting System(s)?

- Who is the supplier of your Image Sharing System(s)?

- Who is the supplier of your Decision Support System(s)?

MU Practice Analysis and Worksheets: You can conduct an eligibility, financial impact, and measure requirement analysis using online tools. To download an analysis worksheet and access the online tools, scan the QR code at the beginning of this chapter or go to **prepare.theMUguide.com.**

Once you've collected answers to the questions above, go to **prepare.theMUguide.com** to calculate your eligibility and the financial impact of the CMS EHR Incentive Programs. Analysis results include provider eligibility, certification preparedness, exclusion opportunities, incentive potential through 2015, penalties through 2019, and potential projected gains and losses for your imaging practice.

What if you are eligible for both versions?

EPs who are eligible for both the Medicare and Medicaid EHR Incentive Programs must choose which incentive program they wish to participate in when they register. Before 2015, any EP may switch programs only once after the first incentive payment is initiated.

Step 3:
Determining your meaningful use measure requirements

In conjunction with determining your eligibility and financial impact, you should also analyze your imaging practice to determine your meaningful use measure requirements and exclusion opportunities. As we've already discussed, the incentive program is based on individual EPs, so all radiologists at your practice may not have the same requirements. For example, if you have a group of 10 radiologists, you really have to look at each radiologist to determine their individual exclusion opportunities.

This assessment of your imaging practice will prove invaluable in determining which of the 25 objectives and measures of the Medicare EHR Incentive Program your practice will need to perform and demonstrate in order to achieve meaningful use. Your group will be able to claim exclusions for several of the 25 measures based on individual EPs meeting exclusion criteria.

In order to complete your online analysis, you must answer the following questions as well as questions outlined in Step 2. Note that a worksheet with all required questions for both Step 2 and Step 3 is available for download from the online companion website. Measures and certification criteria questions include:

• Do you perform Interventional Radiology?

• Do you perform Diagnostic Radiology?

• Do you perform Teleradiology?

• Will you see patients 2 years or older?

• Will you see patients 13 years or older?

• Do you have any patients 65 years or older or 5 years or younger with records maintained using certified EHR technology?

• Will you write more than 100 prescriptions?

• Will you order lab tests whose results are either in a positive/negative or numeric format?

• Will you perform immunizations?

• Will you collect any reportable syndromic information on your patients?

• Do you believe any of the three vital signs (height, weight, and blood pressure) have relevance to your scope of practice?

- Will you be on the receiving end of any transition of care?

- Will you transfer a patient to another setting or refer a patient to another provider?

- Will you perform any office visits?

- Will you receive requests from patients or their agents for an electronic copy of patient health information?

- Are there professional services rendered in your practice where you do not have a physical encounter with your patients (e.g. teleradiology, remote interpretation…)?

> **MU Practice Analysis and Worksheets:** You can conduct a measures and certification criteria analysis to determine potential exclusion opportunities using online tools. To download an analysis worksheet and access the online tools, scan the QR code at the beginning of this chapter or go to **prepare.theMUguide.com.**

While a full practice analysis is necessary to determine the exact measures that individual radiologists will be responsible for reporting, answering the questions above, as well as those in Step 2, and entering your information into the online practice analyzer at **prepare.theMUguide.com** will suggest measures that you may be excluded from reporting.

Potential exclusion opportunities for diagnostic radiologists

Since a high proportion of the radiologists that practice today fall under the classification of diagnostic radiologist, let's examine the potential set of objectives and measures required for this group of EPs. The three lists below outline the 12 potential core and menu set objectives and six CQMs up for consideration for this specific radiology user population after exemptions are taken.

Core Set Objectives:

- **42 CFR §495.6(d)(2):** Implement drug-drug and drug-allergy interaction checks.

- **42 CFR §495.6(d)(3):** Maintain an up-to-date problem list of current and active diagnoses ("seen by the EP" measure; see chapter 7 for guidance).

- **42 CFR §495.6(d)(5):** Maintain active medication list ("seen by the EP" measure; see chapter 7 for guidance).

- **42 CFR §495.6(d)(6):** Maintain active medication allergy list ("seen by the EP" measure; see chapter 7 for guidance).

- **42 CFR §495.6(d)(7):** Record demographics (preferred language, gender, race, ethnicity, date of birth) ("seen by the EP" measure; see chapter 7 for guidance).

- **42 CFR §495.6(d)(9):** Record smoking status for patients 13 years old or older ("seen by the EP" measure; see chapter 7 for guidance).

- **42 CFR §495.6(d)(10):** Report ambulatory clinical quality measures to CMS or the States.

- **42 CFR §495.6(d)(11):** Implement one clinical decision support rule relevant to specialty or high clinical priority along with the ability to track compliance with that rule.

- **42 CFR §495.6(d)(12):** Provide patients with an electronic copy of their health information (including diagnostic test results, problem list, medication list, medication allergies) upon request.

- **42 CFR §495.6(d)(14):** Capability to exchange key clinical information (for example: problem list, medication list, medication allergies, diagnostic test results) among providers of care and patient-authorized entities electronically.

- **42 CFR §495.6(d)(15):** Protect electronic health information created or maintained by the certified EHR technology through the implementation of appropriate technical capabilities.

Menu Set Objectives:

- **42 CFR §495.6(e)(2):** Incorporate clinical lab test results into certified EHR technology as structured data.

Clinical Quality Measures:

- **NFQ 0013 – Hypertension Blood Pressure Measurement:** Percentage of patient visits for patients aged 18 years and older with a diagnosis of hypertension who have been seen for at least 2 office visits, with blood pressure (BP) recorded.

- **NQF 0028 – Tobacco Use Assessment and Cessation Intervention:** (a) Percentage of patients aged 18 years or older who have been seen for at least 2 office visits, who were queried about tobacco use one or more times within 24 months. (b) Percentage of patients aged 18 years and older identified as tobacco users within the past 24 months and have been seen for at least 2 office visits, who received cessation intervention.

- **NQF 0421/PQRI 128 – Adult Weight Screening and Follow-up:** Percentage of patients aged 18 years and older with a calculated BMI in the past six months or during the current visit documented in the medical record and if the most recent BMI is outside parameters, a follow-up plan is documented.

- **NFQ 0043/PQRI 111 – Pneumonia Vaccination Status for Older Adults:** Percentage of patients 65 years of age and older who have ever received pneumococcal vaccine.

- **NQF 0031/PQRI 112 – Breast Cancer Screening:** Percentage of women 40–69 years of age who had a mammogram to screen for breast cancer.

- **NQF 0034/PQRI 113 – Colorectal Cancer Screening:** Percentage of adults 50–75 years of age who had appropriate screening for colorectal cancer.

You will notice that the majority of functionality listed above has the potential to be satisfied by the capabilities of most modern radiology IT systems or practice management solutions. As such, no additional direct radiologist action would be required to satisfy these objectives. For example, the first seven core set objectives and one menu set objective above will most likely be satisfied by certified radiology IT systems. The remaining core set objectives above may be part of your radiology IT systems or patient portal and the final core set objective above will most likely be achievable through nationally implemented decision support standards. The final core set objective in the list above will require an internal audit of your security risks.

Despite the above sample exclusion analysis for this EP classification, you will need to perform an analysis for each radiology EP in your practice in order to fully determine the final set of core and menu set objectives and measures required to achieve meaningful use.

8

CHAPTER 9
Developing Your Meaningful Use Strategy

STEP 4:
Meeting with your practice stakeholders

STEP 5:
Meeting with your radiology IT vendors

Develop your strategy even further.

To further develop your strategy, access additional resources, and download helpful worksheets that support the building of your full meaningful use strategy, scan the QR code above or go to **develop.theMUguide.com.**

In the second chapter of the 10-step approach to achieving meaningful use, we discuss techniques for developing your strategy by meeting with your practice stakeholders and radiology IT vendors.

Step 4:
Meeting with your practice stakeholders

A key step on your path to achieving meaningful use involves not only an analysis of your existing imaging IT environment, but also meeting with the meaningful use stakeholders at your organization. Conducting an infrastructure analysis and working with others at your practice will ensure you have the necessary plans in place to be successful on your journey toward meaningful use. Identify your imaging practice stakeholders and determine if a meaningful use taskforce exists at an institutional level within your organization. If you practice in a hospital setting and a taskforce exists, it is recommended that a representative from your imaging practice join that group. Below are a few tips for meeting with your meaningful use stakeholders based on your practice setting type.

- **Hospital Setting:** It is important for you to understand your institutional plan. If you practice in a hospital setting, it is essential for you to speak with your CIO, CMIO, and any other key individuals that are responsible for meaningful use. You may discover that your EPs are able to leverage your organization's certified EHR technology and combine it with certified imaging technology to achieve meaningful use.

- **Group Practice Setting:** If you work predominately in a group practice setting, speak with your medical director to determine if your group will be participating in the CMS EHR Incentive Programs. Based on this discussion, you will need to ensure your imaging practice has the appropriate mix of certified EHR technology to satisfy all meaningful use measures and objectives.

- **Imaging Center Setting:** If you practice in an imaging center, you will most likely not have a Complete EHR to leverage, so you will need to ensure your group has the appropriate mix of certified EHR technology to satisfy all meaningful use measures and objectives. If you plan to leverage any of your organization's EHR technology, you will need to make sure that you have the necessary integrations in place to transfer information for compliance, monitoring, and attestation purposes.

Consider your practice setting as part of your plan for determining potential solution options. Identifying your patient mix as well as imaging practice scenario allows you to better understand the implications of meaningful use on your individual EPs and group.

IMAGING PRACTICE SETTING CONSIDERATIONS

Practice Setting	Radiologist EP Eligibility	Solution
Inpatient Hospital only (>90% of all business)	No	N/A
Inpatient/Outpatient	Yes (if OP > 10%)	Leverage hospital IT (if hospital >50%)
Inpatient/Imaging Centers	Yes (if IC > 10%)	Leverage hospital IT (if hospital >50%)
Imaging Centers	Yes	Complete radiology IT (single or multi-vendor)
Teleradiology	Variable	Complete radiology IT (single or multi-vendor)

Source: Meaningful Use: The government's billion dollar gift to radiologists. 13 October 2010. Diagnostic Imaging.

Building your meaningful use team

If your group is large, you will want to build a series of meaningful use sub-teams and designate a lead for each functional area. If you are at a smaller practice, it is likely that a small handful of individuals will share these responsibilities. Either way, your core team should schedule routine meetings and develop a clear path with tangible goals and outcomes in mind. The following diagram outlines a sample structure for core and sub-core teams as part of your organization's meaningful use taskforce.

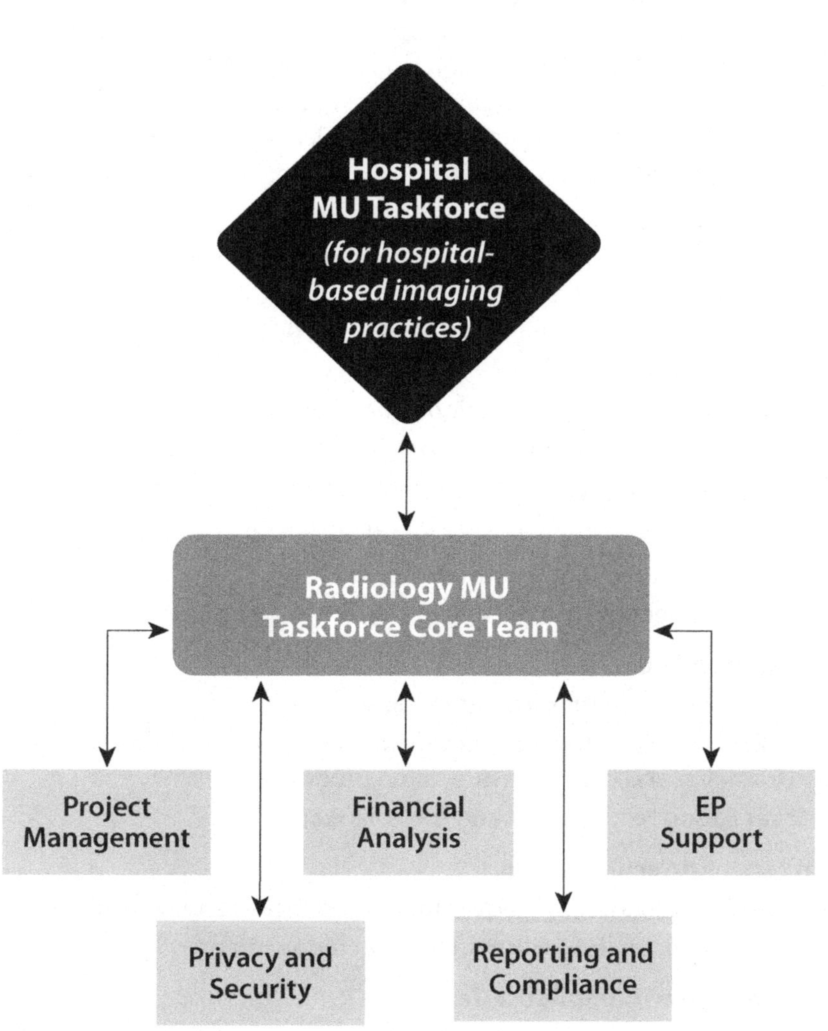

Radiology MU Taskforce Worksheet: Independent of your practice setting type, building your core team for meaningful use will be instrumental to your success. To download the MU taskforce planning worksheet, scan the QR code at the beginning of this chapter or go to **develop.theMUguide.com.**

The **Radiology MU Taskforce Core Team** should provide oversight for all of your imaging practice's meaningful use-related initiatives. For hospital-based practices, this includes participation in facility-wide meaningful use meetings and planning with your organization's core initiatives team. Within your core team, you should consider implementing a plan and creating sub-teams with defined responsibilities.

- **Project Management Team**
  - Develop, implement, and monitor your imaging practice's meaningful use plan.
  - Communicate with radiology IT vendors on technology, certification, reporting, and attestation.
  - Create meaningful use educational materials for EPs, manage upgrades, implementations, and timelines with radiology IT vendors.

- **Financial Analysis Team**
  - Calculate financial impact of meaningful use and make recommendations.
  - Track future stages and financial impact.
  - Monitor projections and incentive payments against plan.

- **EP Support Team**
  - Evaluate and monitor provider readiness.
  - Work with project management team and reporting and compliance team to formalize and deliver an education program to EPs.
  - Act as liaison between EPs and the core team.

- **Privacy and Security Team**
  - Monitor meaningful use requirements and make recommendations.
  - Develop and implement a plan to meet requirements.

- **Reporting and Compliance Team**
  - Create plan for achieving, demonstrating, and reporting meaningful use requirements.
  - Develop reports for EPs.
  - Maintain and sustain program compliance.
  - Contribute to education plan.

Taking the time to plan your strategy and leverage the work being done by others within your organization will enable you to meet all of your meaningful use goals. Collaborating with decision-makers and key users will ensure an easier transition toward meaningful use compliance.

Step 5:
Meeting with your radiology IT vendors

Once you've met with your practice stakeholders and fully understand the meaningful use plans of your organization, you will be ready to meet with your existing radiology IT vendors and the potential IT partners that will help you achieve meaningful use and meet the technological requirements of the program for which your EPs have enrolled. In Step 3, we revealed how a majority of meaningful use measures can be satisfied by many of the current RIS applications if they are certified for meaningful use. It is recommended that you not only enter into discussions with your RIS vendor, but also your PACS, Patient Portal, Image Sharing, and Radiology Reporting vendors and subsequently develop a comprehensive strategy.

Understanding the vendor landscape

Until the Final Rule was released in July 2010, radiology IT vendors did not think that meaningful use applied to them or their customers; a sentiment shared by the entire radiology community. Now that radiology EP eligibility is well established, a variety of diagnostic imaging IT providers are stepping up to the plate. During the second half of 2011, nearly a dozen radiology-specific vendor solutions achieved Modular or Complete EHR certification. Even with the uptick in certified technology for radiology EPs, you need to be cautious as you build your strategy—there is no panacea for tackling this government initiative.

Remember, your imaging practice will need to "possess" EHR technology that has been tested and certified for all 33 Certification Criteria regardless of the exclusions that your EPs claim. When reviewing your strategy against vendor solutions, make certain that the core set measures, menu set measures, and CQMs you select are in fact certified components of the technology you plan to use to demonstrate meaningful use.

Questions to ask your existing and prospective vendors

Once you've identified your primary radiology IT vendors to pursue as part of your strategy for meaningful use, you should schedule a meeting and use the flow chart below as a basis for your conversations with your vendors to assess their plans and better understand their meaningful use road maps.

RADIOLOGY IT VENDOR QUESTIONS

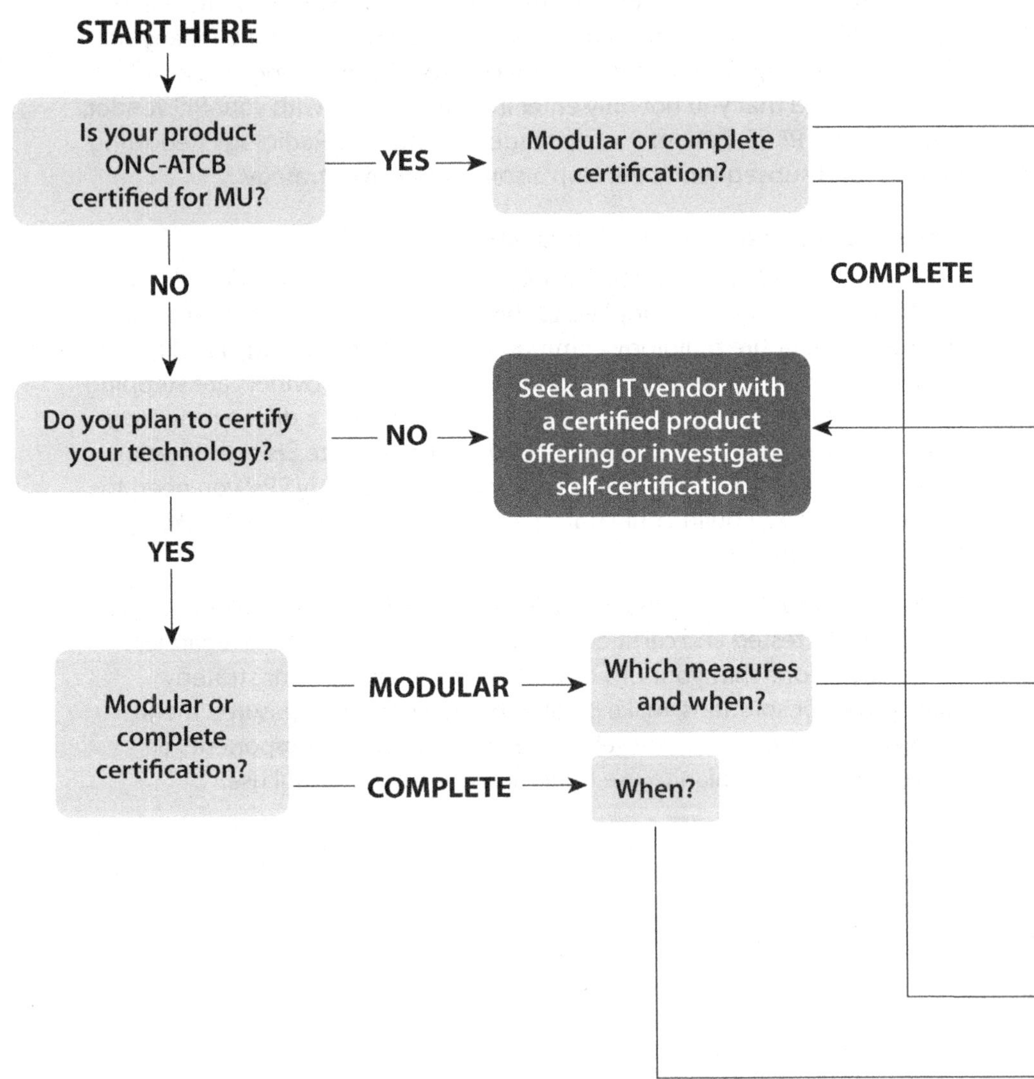

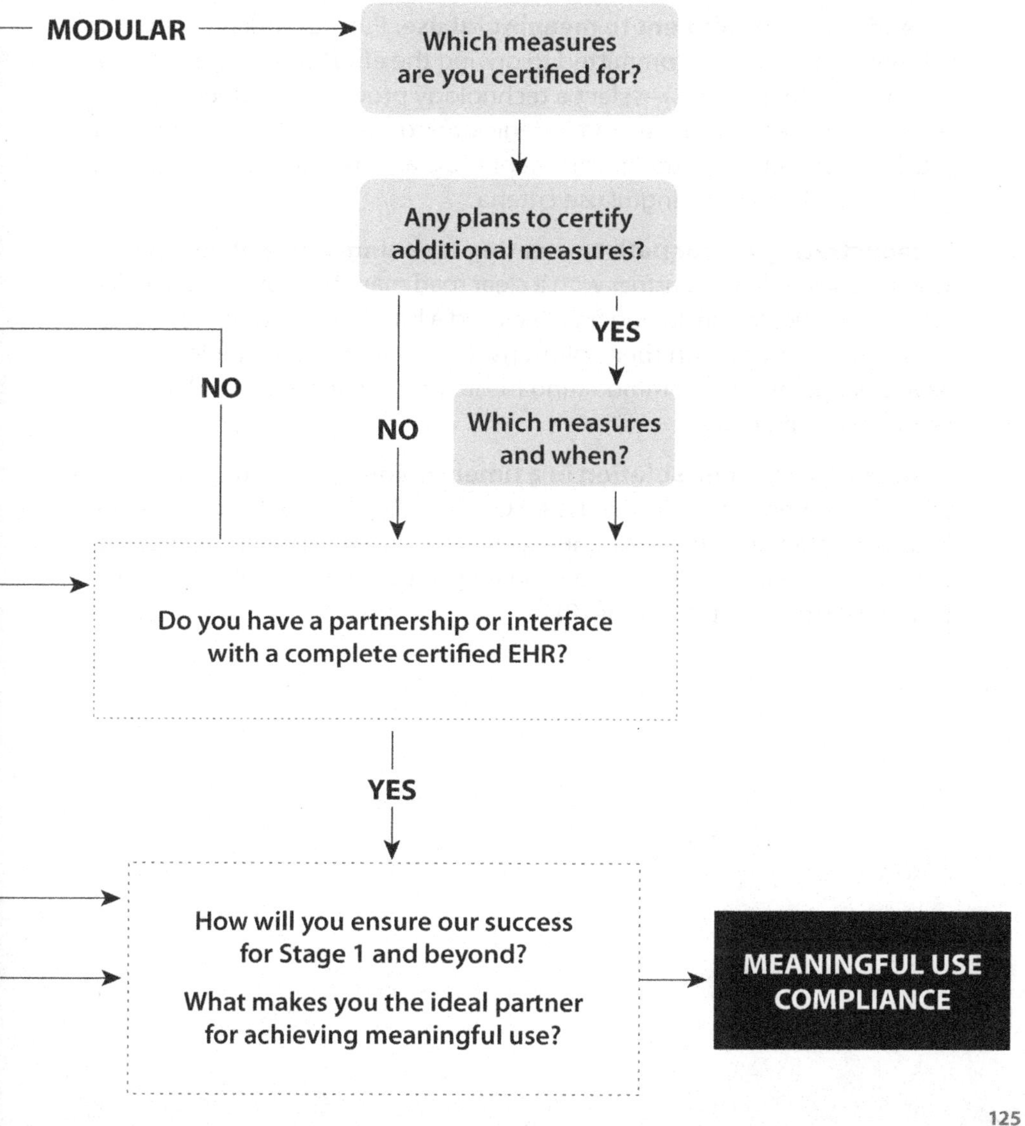
MODULAR
Which measures are you certified for?
Any plans to certify additional measures?
YES
NO
NO
Which measures and when?
Do you have a partnership or interface with a complete certified EHR?
YES
How will you ensure our success for Stage 1 and beyond?
What makes you the ideal partner for achieving meaningful use?
MEANINGFUL USE COMPLIANCE

Seeking the ideal radiology IT vendor partner

Partnering with the right technology provider is critical to the success of your meaningful use project. Seek a technology partner that is committed to providing not only solutions that are certified for the CMS EHR Incentive Programs, but also ones that provide guidance and support to help your organization recognize the impact of the program and better understand what you need to do to successfully roll out your meaningful use strategy.

If you are in the market to replace or upgrade your existing radiology IT infrastructure, you should seek an IT partner who supports your meaningful use strategy by:

- **Extending a commitment to meaningful use.** Pursue working with an IT solution vendor that is committed to driving the effort toward meaningful use for all of their clients—select a technology provider that understands the value of meaningful use and is dedicated to assisting their customers in satisfying objectives of the government program and maintain compliance with the evolving meaningful use criteria.

- **Demonstrating a clear path to meeting meaningful use objectives.** This includes finding a partner with a clear road map that outlines a detailed plan for certification including timelines and a list of meaningful use criteria they plan to satisfy with their solutions. The ideal partner should also have clear plans for accommodating future program changes and future program requirements.

- **Delivering a certified solution in a timely manner.** Your imaging practice will need to begin meaningful use by October 3, 2012 in order to reap the full financial potential of the CMS EHR Incentive Programs. Therefore, the ideal partner should be able to provide and fully implement ONC-ATCB certified technology prior to the end of 2012.

• **Simplifying processes by offering a dedicated services team to support the technology.** Engaging with a software provider that is educated on the topic of meaningful use is key. The optimal partner should have experience in assisting clients understand, apply for, and successfully demonstrate meaningful use of certified EHR technology. They should be agile and have a proactive plan in place to provide continued support and updates as federal regulations evolve.

• **Providing flexibility to integrate certified solutions with existing technology and workflows.** Seek a provider that offers flexible solutions to provide minimal impact and disruption to your existing workflows. This includes integrating the technology with your existing solutions and providing effective communication with other systems.

Meaningful use is a long-term strategy and the ideal IT provider is one that you can develop a "true" partnership with to ensure alignment with your meaningful use goals and objectives. Taking the time to evaluate your solution providers and their technology will be instrumental to your success with the program.

9

CHAPTER 10
Executing Your Meaningful Use Strategy

STEP 6:
Planning your meaningful use technological
and operational strategies

STEP 7:
Acquiring and implementing certified
EHR technology

Get additional support for executing your strategy.

To access additional information and updated resources related to planning and executing
your operational and technical strategy and implementing certified EHR technology, scan
the QR code above or go to **execute.theMUguide.com.**

In this third chapter of the 10-step approach to achieving meaningful use, we discuss techniques for executing your strategy through planning your technological and operational strategies and acquiring and implementing certified technology.

Step 6:
Planning your meaningful use technological and operational strategies

The steps leading up to your operational planning will probably not require outside assistance. However, this is the point in the 10-step approach that you begin to spend money and implement your strategy, and it is also the point at which your existing workflow and processes may potentially be impacted. As a result, Step 6 is the first time in the process that it may be appropriate to seek consultative assistance.

There are a number of meaningful use consultants in the field ranging from full-service agencies to smaller, specialized meaningful use consulting service providers. Many of these consulting firms offer services that help align your performance improvement objectives with your technical and operational goals. Consultative assistance can be beneficial for budget preparation, workflow documentation, technical specifications and analysis, connectivity and data exchange, defining vendor and technology requirements, and reviewing your existing IT infrastructure.

In addition to consultants, Regional Extension Centers (RECs) have been established to help EPs as they tackle meaningful use. While the RECs target their assistance to eligible primary care providers in smaller practices, they also serve as resources for all providers in a given geographic region. We provide a full list of RECs and additional information in chapter 17.

Whether you decide to use outside services, an REC, or plan your technological and operational strategy internally, the key objective of your planning efforts should be to minimize radiology EP workflow burden. You will need to determine how much technology is required to make certain that your EPs do not have to perform unnecessary duplicate entry or redundant data capture.

A good example might be if your imaging practice needs to measure blood pressure. The questions you need to ask yourself and others in your group include:

• Who captures this information? The radiologist? The technologist? Other clinical staff?

• How does this information get entered?

• Where does it happen, and when does it happen?

• Once data is collected, how is it shared and reported?

Allocating resources and clearly defining clinical and administrative staff responsibilities for meaningful use will be critical to your success. Leveraging your care team, practice staff, informatics leads, administrators, and your radiology EPs will be instrumental in planning and implementing the various aspects of your meaningful use operational and technical strategy.

Step 7:
Acquiring and implementing certified EHR technology

Once you have determined your operational and technological requirements, you may need to acquire or implement certified EHR technology to comply with program requirements not satisfied by your existing technology. This involves considering potential upgrades or add-ons to your RIS, PACS, practice management system, and any other IT platform that may be used to demonstrate meaningful use. Also, it is important that your practice has access to a meaningful use dashboard so that your group can view and track all of your individual EP meaningful use measures to ensure ongoing compliance. This functionality might be provided by one of your existing systems or may require implementation of a separate dashboard application.

Since you have to monitor each EP separately, and have so many measures to keep track of, you will need a central system to monitor all of your EP activity, across all patients, for each radiologist in your imaging practice. A dashboard allows your senior administrators or individual EPs to check their compliance status for a given attestation period. It also provides a record of individual EP activity, which may prove helpful in the event of an audit.

As part of building your technology acquisition and upgrade plan, you will need to conduct product certification status checks. Don't forget that product certification is specific to both a vendor's product and its specific version. In other words, you may need to upgrade your technology to a newer version of software from your IT vendor in order to meet the certified EHR technology requirement.

In chapter 6, we briefly discussed the Certified HIT Product List (CHPL). It's at this stage that the CHPL is an excellent resource for searching certified EHR technology by product name, vendor name, CHPL number (if known) or specific certification criteria met. This authoritative and comprehensive listing of certified Complete EHRs and EHR Modules offers a certification summary bar and shopping cart to aid in your certified technology search.

ONC Certified HIT Product List (CHPL): The CHPL provides a fully searchable catalog of products certified for meaningful use. To find out more about the CHPL website, scan the QR code at the beginning of this chapter or go to **execute.theMUguide.com.**

Hospital-based radiology practice: Complete Certified EHR/RIS

Now let's apply what we discussed above to a typical hospital-based radiology practice with a complete certified EHR or RIS. The diagram below depicts the various integrations and flow of information present in this type of practice environment. Connected to the complete certified EHR/RIS is a meaningful use data aggregation system that feeds information and data into an EP dashboard. This dashboard can be made available to staff EPs and radiology EPs and can be used for reporting meaningful use measures to CMS for attestation.

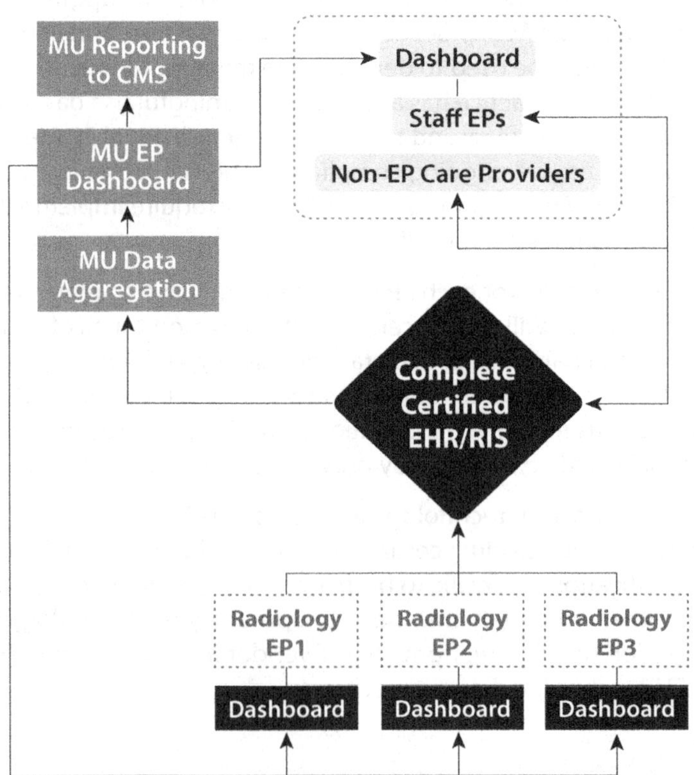

Hospital-based radiology practice: combined Certified EHR with separate RIS

For hospital-based radiology practices with combined certified EHR technology and a separate RIS, the environment is slightly different. In this case, the EP dashboard can be presented to staff EPs, but the dashboard is not able to be presented directly to the radiology EPs because their workflow is conducted through the RIS. With this separation in place, the dashboards cannot be made available for viewing by the radiologists unless the interfaces are in place to carry the pertinent data through the system.

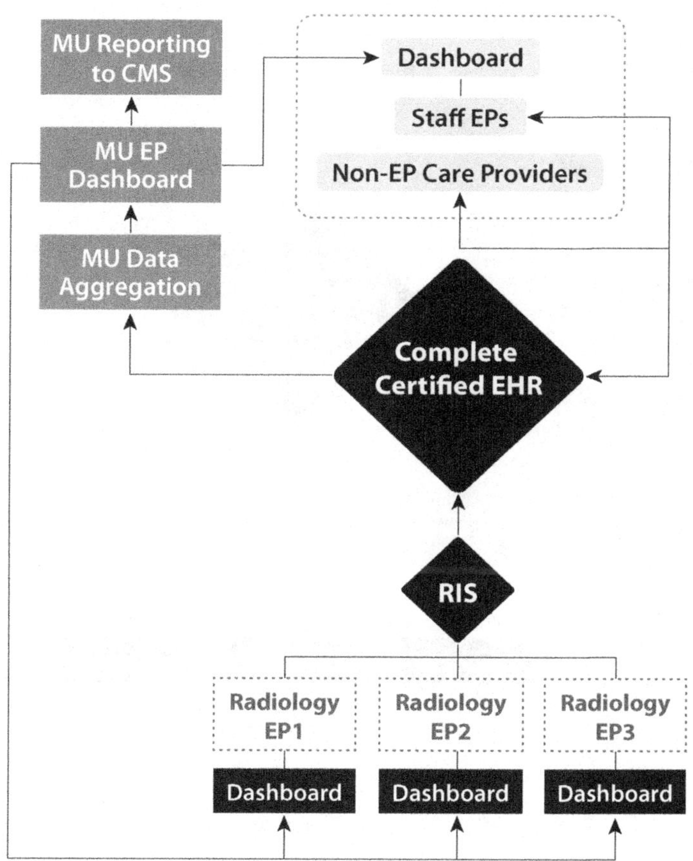

Non-hospital based radiology practice: Complete Certified RIS

In this setting, we will examine the various integrations and flow of information present at a non-hospital based radiology practice with a complete certified RIS. In this scenario, the complete certified RIS pushes data to a non-certified information system. With the complete certified RIS present, data is sent to a meaningful use data aggregation system that feeds information and data into an EP dashboard that can be made available to the radiologists. This data aggregation system is also used to report measures to CMS for attestation.

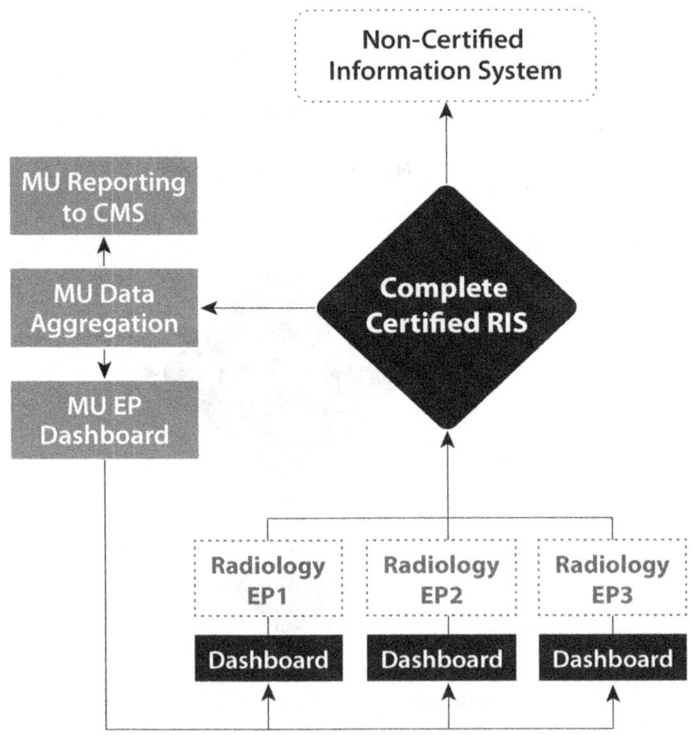

Non-hospital based radiology practice: Modular Certified RIS with possessed Complete EHR

Next, let's assess the situation at a non-hospital based radiology practice with a modular certified RIS and possession of a complete certified EHR. In this instance, the modular certified RIS pushes data to a non-certified information system. With the modular certified RIS present, data is sent to a meaningful use data aggregation system that feeds information and data into an EP dashboard that can be made available to the radiologists. This data aggregation system is also used to report measures to CMS for attestation. The possession of a complete certified EHR is key to fulfilling program requirements.

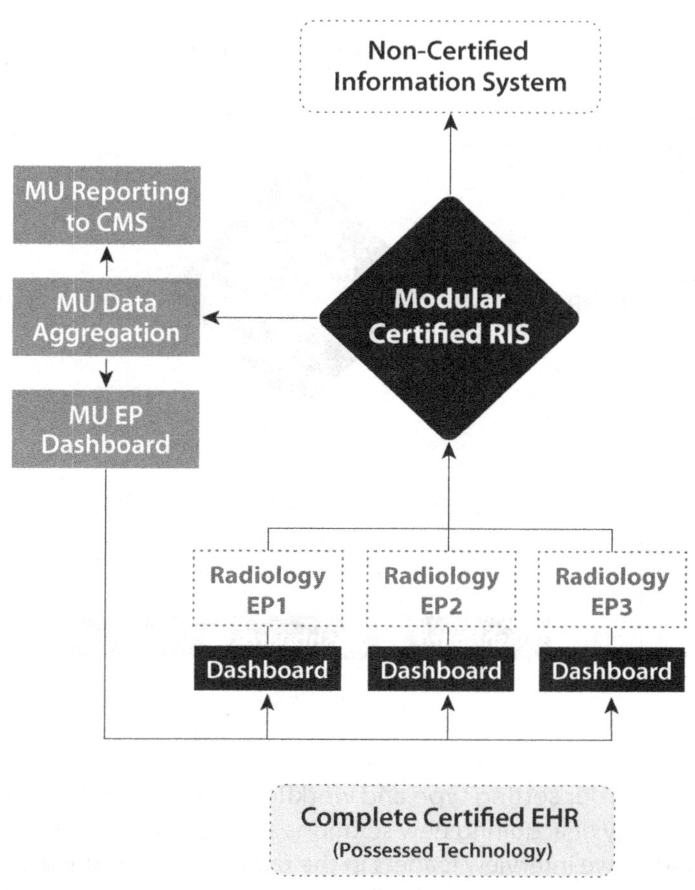

Non-hospital based radiology practice: Modular Certified RIS with separate Complete EHR

For this final scenario, we take a look at a non-hospital based radiology practice with a modular certified RIS and separate complete certified EHR solution. This is similar to the previous scenario, except now your imaging practice is engaging the certified EHR and pushing your EP's non-excluded measures from your modular certified RIS to your EHR via an electronic interface. This workflow eliminates duplicate data entry and allows your group to take advantage of the complete certified EHRs meaningful use data aggregation system to feed information and data into an EP dashboard that can be made available to your radiologists. As with the other practice setting scenarios, the data aggregation system can be used to report measures to CMS for attestation.

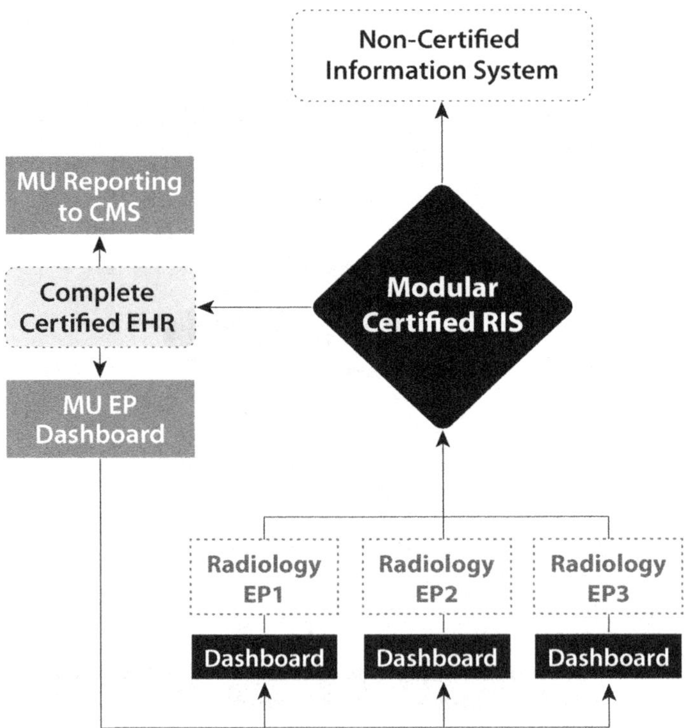

Take into account your setting type and workflows when upgrading your existing technology or acquiring new solutions as part of your meaningful use strategy. In Part III, we interview leaders in the radiology community and learn from them as they discuss ways in which they are approaching certified EHR technology requirements for their practices.

10

CHAPTER 11
Sustaining Your Meaningful Use Strategy

STEP 8:
Registering online with CMS

STEP 9:
Monitoring your meaningful use compliance regularly

STEP 10:
Attesting online with CMS

More information to help you sustain your strategy.

To access video links, download useful program worksheets, and get even more
assistance during the final steps in demonstrating and achieving meaningful use
success, scan the QR code above or go to **sustain.theMUguide.com.**

In this fourth and final chapter of the 10-step approach to achieving meaningful use for radiology EPs, we discuss the requirements for sustaining your strategy through online registration with CMS, regular compliance monitoring, and the reporting period attestation process.

Step 8:
Registering online with CMS

Once you've determined your imaging practice's eligibility for the CMS EHR Incentive Programs, each EP will need to register online using the Medicare and Medicaid EHR Incentive Programs Registration and Attestation System. Registration must be completed prior to submitting meaningful use attestation. Even though registration and attestation can occur at the same time, it is advisable not to wait until your practice is ready to attest to register for the program. While an EP can register prior to possessing all necessary certified EHR technology, this information is required before an EP can attest.

All EPs applying under the Medicare version of the program are required to have a National Provider Identifier (NPI) and Nation Plan and Provider Enumeration System (NPPES) account. All EPs will also need to be enrolled in the Provider Enrollment, Chain and Ownership System (PECOS). You can check the enrollment status of an EP, and if needed, enroll in the system, via the CMS EHR Incentive Programs website.

CMS also allows EPs to designate a third party to register and attest on their behalf. If an EP or imaging practice chooses to do so, the individuals performing these tasks will need to have an Identity and Access Management System (I&A) account and must be associated with each EP and their NPI. If the user working on behalf of your EPs does not have an account, one can be obtained via the I&A Security Check on the program's official website.

MU Registration Process

The meaningful use program registration process for EPs is straightforward and on average takes fifteen to twenty minutes per EP. Once an EP has all of the required accounts setup, they must complete a three-piece questionnaire to successfully register for the program.

- First, the EP will be required to select the version of the program for which they are applying. In the case of eligible radiologists, the majority will select the Medicare version. EPs that are eligible for both versions of the program must choose which incentive program they wish to participate in at this point. Before 2015, an EP may switch programs only once after the first incentive payment is issued.

- Next, the EP will need to select their physician type. For radiology professionals, most EPs will select Doctor of Medicine or Osteopathy.

- The initial registration survey also asks if the registering EP is currently using a certified EHR and to supply the certified EHR number. While this is not a mandatory requirement for registration, the EP will need to provide this information prior to submitting attestation.

- EP name and identifier information is recorded under personal information and is automatically retrieved from the EP's NPI record. At this stage, an EP must also choose the Payee TIN Type. If the payments are to be sent to the EP directly, they will choose the SSN option. If the payments should be sent to an imaging practice or group associated with the EP, the EIN option will be selected. Based on selection, additional details may be required.

- Like the EP's personal information, the practice address and contact details associated with the EP will be automatically populated from the NPI record.

- Once this information is entered, the EP will have an opportunity to verify their registration submission. After verifying that all of the information is correct, the EP must review and agree to a legal notice before their registration can be submitted.

- Once the disclaimer is accepted, the registration website will notify the EP of successful registration if the registration passes all validations. Since the EP will not receive an email confirmation, the EP should record their registration ID and print a copy of the submission receipt page.

Official EP Registration User Guide: CMS has released a step-by-step guide for EPs participating in the Medicare EHR Incentive Program. To download the official registration guide and other helpful information, scan the QR code at the beginning of this chapter or go to **sustain.theMUguide.com**.

Step 9:
Monitoring your meaningful use compliance regularly

Once you have your meaningful use infrastructure up and running, you will need to regularly monitor your compliance against each individual EP's incentive program requirements. This includes implementing a tracking mechanism or dashboard and monitoring the individual EP and group level statuses that we discussed in chapter 10.

The supplier of your certified EHR technology will provide compliance dashboards for your group. In the case of a modular approach to meaningful use, you may be required to implement a third-party solution that aggregates the data from these individual systems. At a minimum, the dashboards that you implement for meaningful use will need to track and allow for reporting by individual EP, facility/location, and date range as well as numerator and denominator for those measures that require such information be reported. It is important to possess a dashboard that generates this data in a format that provides all pertinent information required for attestation. Keep in mind that you will need to track compliance for each individual EP in your practice group.

Note: Each radiology EP is required to attest individually. Make sure that your compliance reporting system provides access to reports for each individual radiology EP in your practice that is participating in the incentive program.

In year one, EPs are only required to report ninety days of data, but if an EP fails even one measure, they will have to begin the ninety-day period for attestation again. As this process will be new to your imaging practice, it is recommended that you monitor your radiology EP compliance on a daily basis so that you have ample time to correct any issues should they arise. Keep these tips in mind as you plan for and approach the attestation process.

Step 10:
Attesting online with CMS

Attestation, or the process of legally stating to CMS that an EP has demonstrated meaningful use of certified EHR technology, is the final step in our 10-step process. Attestation is conducted using the same system that is used for registration—the Medicare and Medicaid EHR Incentive Programs Registration and Attestation System. Prior to attesting as an EP under the Medicare program, you will need to have:

• Determined your eligibility to participate in the Medicare program.

• Successfully registered for the Medicare program on the CMS EHR Incentive Programs Registration System.

• Met the required number of core set, menu set, and clinical quality measures.

• Recorded meeting your meaningful use criteria for the appropriate time period.

> **CMS EHR Attestation Calculator:** Prior to beginning the attestation process, you can check EP compliance with having met all program requirements to successfully complete attestation. To access the CMS EP Meaningful Use Calculator, scan the QR code at the beginning of this chapter or go to **sustain.theMUguide.com.**

MU Attestation Process

Similar in look and feel to the registration pages, the attestation process guides the EP or designated third party through a series of topics including attestation information, core measures, menu measures, core CQMs, alternate core CQMs, and discretionary CQMs. The attestation process is as follows:

• First, the EP will need to provide basic attestation information to begin the process. This includes an EHR Certification Number, reporting period start date and reporting period end date. For the first year, the reporting period must be a minimum of ninety consecutive days. For each subsequent year, the attestation period must be 365 days (or 366 in a leap year like 2012). It is important to note that the CMS EHR Certification Number (which is 15 alphanumeric characters) is different than the ONC CHPL Product Number issued to the EP's technology provider.

- Next, the EP will need to complete all fifteen questions in the core measures section. Each question is unique, but may potentially require entry of patient record details, exemptions, and numerators/denominators if exclusion criteria are not met. Pay special attention to questionnaire 10—the EP will need to indicate if they will report CQMs to CMS in the manner specified by CMS. If the EP answers "no" to this question, the EP will not receive payment.

- After completing the core measures section, the EP will need to complete the menu set measures section. The first screen provides a comprehensive list of all 10 measures and allows the EP to select their five menu measures for reporting, one of which must be from the public health section (even if an exclusion applies). The EP will then be asked to provide criteria for each menu measure that is selected.

- The next section contains the CQM questionnaires. First, the EP will need to input data related to all three core or alternate core CQMs. After completing all required core/alternate core measures, the EP will need to select three additional measures to report to CMS. You will recall that in chapter 4 we discussed measures that are relevant to the radiology community. While your measure selections may vary, the attestation system requires that denominators, numerators, and exclusions be entered for each additional measure that is selected.

- Upon completion of all sections, the EP may proceed to the attestation summary page. Here the EP can review and change the core, menu, and CQMs that were entered in the questionnaire sections.

- Finally, the EP is required to agree to a series of statements related to the authenticity and accuracy of their attestation. Upon agreeing with all statements, the EP is directed to a confirmation page. After ensuring the information is correct, an attestation disclaimer is presented to the EP. Upon agreeing with this final disclaimer, the EP's attestation will be submitted and the system accepts or rejects the submission. Once accepted, the EP will qualify for an incentive payment for the reporting period and receive payment approximately four to eight weeks after successful submission.

- If the EP attestation is rejected, you may contact your Regional Extension Center (REC) for guidance. We review RECs and provide a full list of current centers in chapter 17 of this guide.

Methods for calculating measures

For EPs, there are a few ways of measuring compliance based on calculation requirements for each specific core and menu set objective. The three types of reporting requirements include measures with a denominator of unique patients regardless of whether the patient's records are maintained using certified EHR technology, measures with a denominator based on counting actions for patients whose records are maintained using certified EHR technology, and measures requiring only a yes/no attestation.

The following objectives have associated measures with a denominator of unique patients regardless of whether the patient's records are maintained using certified EHR technology:

- **42 CFR §495.6(d)(3):** Maintain an up-to-date problem list of current and active diagnoses.

- **42 CFR §495.6(d)(5):** Maintain active medication list.

- **42 CFR §495.6(d)(6):** Maintain active medication allergy list.

- **42 CFR §495.6(d)(7):** Record demographics: preferred language, gender, race, ethnicity, date of birth.

- **42 CFR §495.6(e)(5):** Provide patients with timely electronic access to their health information (including lab results, problem list, medication list, medication allergies) within four business days of the information being available to the EP.

- **42 CFR §495.6(e)(6):** Use certified EHR technology to identify patient-specific education resources and provide those resources to the patient if appropriate.

The following objectives have associated measures with a denominator based on counting actions for patients whose records are maintained using certified EHR technology:

- **42 CFR §495.6(d)(1):** Use computerized provider order entry (CPOE) for medication orders directly entered by any licensed health care professional who can enter orders into the medical record per state, local, and professional guidelines.

- **42 CFR §495.6(d)(4):** Generate and transmit permissible prescriptions electronically (eRx).

- **42 CFR §495.6(d)(8):** Record and chart changes in vital signs: height, weight, blood pressure; calculate and display BMI; plot and display growth charts for children 2–20 years (including BMI).

- **42 CFR §495.6(d)(9):** Record smoking status for patients 13 years old or older.

- **42 CFR §495.6(e)(2):** Incorporate clinical lab test results into certified EHR technology as structured data.

- **42 CFR §495.6(d)(12):** Provide patients with an electronic copy of their health information (including diagnostic test results, problem list, medication list, medication allergies) upon request.

- **42 CFR §495.6(d)(13):** Provide clinical summaries for patients for each office visit.

- **42 CFR §495.6(e)(4):** Send reminders to patients per patient preference for preventive/follow-up care.

- **42 CFR §495.6(e)(7):** The EP who receives a patient from another setting of care or provider of care or believes an encounter is relevant should perform medication reconciliation.

- **42 CFR §495.6(e)(8):** The EP who transitions their patient to another setting of care or provider of care or refers their patient to another provider of care should provide summary of care record for each transition of care or referral.

The following objectives have associated measures requiring only a yes/no attestation:

- **42 CFR §495.6(d)(2):** Implement drug-drug and drug-allergy interaction checks.

- **42 CFR §495.6(e)(1):** Implement drug-formulary checks.

- **42 CFR §495.6(e)(3):** Generate lists of patients by specific conditions to use for quality improvement, reduction of disparities, research or outreach.

- **42 CFR §495.6(d)(11):** Implement one clinical decision support rule relevant to specialty or high clinical priority along with the ability to track compliance with that rule.

- **42 CFR §495.6(d)(14):** Capability to exchange key clinical information (for example: problem list, medication list, medication allergies, diagnostic test results) among providers of care and patient-authorized entities electronically.

- **42 CFR §495.6(e)(9):** Capability to submit electronic data to immunization registries or Immunization Information Systems and actual submission in accordance with applicable law and practice.

- **42 CFR §495.6(e)(10):** Capability to submit electronic syndromic surveillance data to public health agencies and actual submission in accordance with applicable law and practice.

- **42 CFR §495.6(d)(15):** Protect electronic health information created or maintained by the certified EHR technology through the implementation of appropriate technical capabilities.

These measure-type groups were designed to reduce the burden on providers. For more information about the various types of measure groupings, refer to the incentive programs Final Rule (FR 75 44376 – 44380).

Risks, audits, and record keeping

According to documentation in the CMS Final Rule, one commenter expressed a concern that "attestation is an insufficient means to hold providers accountable for the expenditure of public funds and to protect against fraud and abuse." CMS shares the concern for potential fraud and abuse and has developed an audit strategy to address these types of risks. With that said, any EP attesting to receive an incentive payment under the program may be subject to an audit by the government.

While there are some requirements, like the fact that providers participating in the incentive programs must retain all documentation that supports their demonstration of meaningful use for six years after attestation, EPs can do more to prepare by managing the additional risks associated with attestation. Aside from retaining paper and electronic versions of core and menu set records, cost reports, payment calculations, and CQM documentation, imaging practices can implement a formal risk analysis process, follow existing security and privacy standards, as well as demonstrate due diligence in risk identification and implementation.

Part III:
IMAGING PROVIDER PERSPECTIVES

In this third section, we hear from your radiology colleagues as they tackle meaningful use and discuss their experiences along the way. Part III presents a series of in-depth interviews with various leaders—from different practice types and with varying roles and responsibilities—in the radiology community. These "lessons learned" provide invaluable insight into what others are facing as they strategically approach the CMS EHR Incentive Programs and demonstrate meaningful use.

CHAPTER 12
A Conversation with Dr. Keith J. Dreyer

In this chapter, Dr. Keith J. Dreyer, Vice Chairman of Radiology Informatics, Massachusetts General Hospital, offers insight on learning the basics of the CMS EHR Incentive Programs, discusses meaningful use requirements and stakeholder meetings, reviews technical and operational strategies, and comments on the processes that surround meaningful use for radiologists.

About Dr. Keith J. Dreyer

Keith J. Dreyer, DO, PhD, FSIIM

*Vice Chairman of Radiology Informatics, Massachusetts General Hospital
Corporate Director, Enterprise Medical Imaging, Partners Healthcare
Chairman, ACR, IT Government Relations Committee*

Dr. Keith J. Dreyer is the Vice Chairman of Radiology Informatics at Massachusetts General Hospital and Assistant Professor of Radiology at the Harvard Medical School. He is a board-certified diagnostic radiologist and has held his current positions for more than fifteen years. Widely published, he is a leading expert in the field of healthcare information technology including the areas of RIS/PACS, speech recognition, medical imaging distribution, mobile imaging informatics, and electronic health records.

Nationally, Dr. Dreyer holds, and has held, multiple leadership and advisory positions with the American College of Radiology (ACR), American Board of Radiologists (ABR), Radiological Society of North America (RSNA), and the Society for Imaging Informatics in Medicine (SIIM). As the current Co-Chair of the ACR's Information Technology and Informatics Committee, he is actively engaged in federal policy issues and programs including electronic health records, meaningful use, accountable care organizations, and clinical decision support for imaging utilization management. In 2010, Dr. Dreyer facilitated a common vision across all of the major medical imaging organizations for the guidance of federal and state legislations, practice guidelines, and technical specifications. In addition to his industry leadership role, he also serves as a clinical and technical advisor to a number of international medical imaging corporations.

A conversation on meaningful use

What have you and your organization done to educate yourselves on the fundamentals of meaningful use?

Dreyer: Our CIO introduced me to meaningful use during a presentation in late 2009. I asked if there was a plan to include the radiology department and quickly learned that our team needed to educate ourselves on the ins and outs of the program. We reviewed the literature, examined the timetables, analyzed the standards, implementation specifications, and certification criteria, and assessed the reporting requirements. We also used many of the resources on the CMS EHR Incentive Programs website—fact sheets, summaries, and online video tutorials—to better understand meaningful use and build our strategy.

What steps have you taken to determine your eligibility and the financial impact of the CMS EHR Incentive Programs on your imaging practice?

Dreyer: Our group decided to run the practice analyzer at radiologyMU.org as our first step toward determining eligibility and financial impact of the incentive program. We plugged in the numbers for our 250 radiologists and found out that the majority of them were in fact eligible and significant dollars were at stake under the program. Some of the questions that we asked ourselves were:

• Do our radiologists read cases in the hospital setting or ER setting?

• Do they read enough CMS volume?

• How much of the problem for eligibility would we solve if we focused on leveraging certified technology from the hospital?

After reviewing our analysis and the financials, we opted to leverage our hospital's certified EHR technology for meaningful use.

Have you determined your meaningful use measure requirements? If so, what did you discover during that process?

Dreyer: Again, we used the practice analyzer at radiologyMU.org to begin identifying exclusion opportunities. We segmented our radiology practice into diagnostic, interventional, mammography, and teleradiology. This segmentation allowed us to determine the required measures for each radiology EP in our imaging practice.

Have you met with the meaningful use stakeholders at your organization? What can you tell us about that?

Dreyer: At our organization, we have a team that is responsible for certifying our in-house EHR technology and we discussed with them how radiology IT would integrate with that solution. We have also conducted several meetings with our CMO and deputy CMO, who have been assigned to meaningful use. Our primary discussions have included a demonstration of analysis and the justification for including our group in the program. We also met with our CIO, who oversees much of this activity. During the meetings, we reviewed such topics as system integrations, workflows, attestation requirements, and overall technical and operational logistics.

Have you met with your radiology IT vendors? What can you tell us about that?

Dreyer: We have had meetings and discussions with most of our radiology IT providers, but ultimately decided that we would utilize our RIS for meaningful use. We encouraged our RIS vendor to provide at least a modular-certified solution so that when we do integrate with our hospital's complete EHR we will possess a certified chain of connectivity across the organization. One of the primary reasons for requesting this certification from our RIS vendor was to ensure that our radiology solution would meet all of the security and privacy measures associated with the CMS EHR Incentive Programs.

What have you and your organization done to plan your meaningful use technical and operational strategy?

Dreyer: We made the decision early on to go with the hospital and their pathway toward providing technology to staff EPs. Once our plan was in place, the focus shifted to integrating the hospital technology with our radiology department's technology. Part of what we discovered was that we did not need to move this data that tracked radiologist/patient encounters to our EHR; we needed to move that data to our attestation system and meaningful use dashboard, which is the integration we are actively working on completing.

Does your organization plan to acquire and implement new technology to achieve meaningful use? If yes, what type of technology?

Dreyer: I think we are bit unique in that we develop most of the technology we use in our practice. As for new technology, we are designing and developing our attestation system and meaningful use dashboards. Also, our radiology group is responsible for the integration between the RIS and EHR so that we can track patients and accurately measure the reporting requirement for each EP. So for us, it's all about developing the tools that we need to make our existing technology meet the program requirements.

Do you have any comments about the online registration process with CMS?

Dreyer: It's fairly straightforward. CMS added the ability for authorized parties to register on behalf of the individual EPs. Since all of our processes—licensing, accreditation, malpractice, and other activities—are done centrally through administration, it is now much easier for an imaging group like ours to register for the program.

What are your plans to monitor your imaging practice's meaningful use compliance?

Dreyer: Our hospital IT team has already designed the meaningful use dashboards and the attestation system that we plan to use. We also have the ability to track patients that have had an encounter; in radiology this is really considered an interpretation. We have yet to deploy the dashboards as we are deciding on final authorization and access levels for the various stakeholders, department heads, and chairs.

Do you have any comments about the attestation process?

Dreyer: We have not yet attested, but the demo system on the CMS website provides a "feel" for the experience and it appears fairly straightforward. We do know that attestation is currently a manual process, but will be automated within the next few years. When automation becomes available, we plan to link our attestation system with the online system provided by CMS.

Now that we've been through all that… what's next?

Dreyer: We plan to begin demonstrating meaningful use before the end of 2012.

Any final thoughts or advice you would offer to other imaging providers that are developing their strategies for meaningful use? Any thoughts or hopes for future stages of the program?

Dreyer: It helps a lot to understand the fundamentals of the program and run an analysis for your imaging practice. It's well known that most radiologists are eligible, so the question really becomes whether or not you want to participate. Next, you need to review your measure requirements and make sure that your IT vendors are prepared to support your strategy. Lastly, I would encourage you to continue reading articles, visiting the official program websites, attending tradeshows, participating in meaningful use lectures, and doing all you can to stay on top of meaningful use as it applies to radiology.

As for future stages, the hope would be that the challenges for medical specialists—lack of direct clinical relevance, access to technology and data, and inflexible requirements—would be better addressed. The incorporation of imaging data as part of meaningful use and specialty-specific requirements would also increase the relevance of the program.

CHAPTER 13
A Conversation with Dr. Alberto F. Goldszal

In this chapter, Dr. Alberto F. Goldszal, CIO, University Radiology Group, offers insight on learning the basics of the CMS EHR Incentive Programs, discusses meaningful use requirements and stakeholder meetings, reviews technical and operational strategies, and comments on the processes that surround meaningful use for radiologists.

About Dr. Alberto F. Goldszal

Alberto F. Goldszal, PhD

Chief Information Officer, University Radiology Group
Adjunct Assistant Professor, Robert Wood Johnson Medical School

Dr. Alberto F. Goldszal has served as the University Radiology Group's Chief Information Officer since 2007. He is responsible for the group's overall informatics strategy and for the implementation of its IT operational goals. His previous positions include Chief Information Officer at Penn Radiology and Chief Information Officer at the NIH's Imaging Sciences Institute. Dr. Goldszal has more than twenty years of experience and expertise in medical informatics, management of healthcare IT organizations, and the implementation and operation of enterprise-wide medical information systems such as RIS/HIS, PACS, teleradiology systems, CPOE, EMRs, and HIEs.

Dr. Goldszal also serves as an Adjunct Assistant Professor of Radiology at the Robert Wood Johnson Medical School, UMDNJ. He has held faculty appointments at the University of Pennsylvania, at the Johns Hopkins University, and at the National Institute of Neurological Disorders and Stroke (NINDS). He is the author of several peer-reviewed publications, book chapters, and abstracts. His professional affiliations include IEEE, AAAS, RSNA, and SIIM. Training credentials include a PhD in Biomedical Engineering from Drexel University and a masters in the Management of Technology at Penn Engineering and at the Wharton Business School of the University of Pennsylvania.

A conversation on meaningful use

What have you and your organization done to educate yourselves on the fundamentals of meaningful use?

Goldszal: First, let me say that it's important to start educating yourself now if you haven't done so already. To educate ourselves on meaningful use we used three primary sources. First, we looked at the basics and general requirements of the program. We attended conferences and lectures and read through various publications. We also relied heavily on word-of-mouth. A second source that we tapped for information was radiologyMU.org. We used this website to better understand the layers under the program as they relate to the medical imaging community—this was invaluable. Lastly, we learned a lot from our RIS vendor, who understood the incentive programs and engaged us early on in the process.

What steps have you taken to determine your eligibility and the financial impact of the CMS EHR Incentive Programs on your imaging practice?

Goldszal: Once you have a good feel for the basics, you need to determine your eligibility and what the program means to your practice from a financial standpoint. The fact that more than 90 percent of all radiologists are eligible for the program means that you are most likely eligible. Even so, you still need to do some simple math to verify that you fall within this group. And the criteria are clear. Like our group, you can apply rules directly from the regulations to determine your eligibility for the program.

First, you need to make sure that your radiologists perform more than 10 percent of their interpretations in an outpatient setting. That's very clear and easy to report on. If you pass that threshold, then you need to look at your practice setting. If you practice in multiple locations like our group does, you need to make sure that more than 50 percent of your outpatient encounters come from a setting that is using certified EHR technology. Again, another simple rule to apply and one with no room for interpretation. Lastly, for the Medicare version of the program, you need to treat Medicare patients and bill for Part B services on the Medicare Physician Fee Schedule in order to be eligible for incentive payments. If you pass those simple tests, you are eligible.

As for the potential financial upside, we did a simple calculation with the number of radiologists in our practice that are eligible and multiplied that by the available incentives over the life of the program. When calculating this potential upside, don't forget that incentives cannot exceed 75 percent of an EP's Medicare Physician Fee Schedule compensation for a given year.

Have you determined your meaningful use measure requirements? If so, what did you discover during that process?

Goldszal: Yes, we have already determined our exclusions and measures for the program. I'll start by saying that there is no question that this step in the process involves work. While there are certain measures that you can pick and choose, there are measures that you cannot avoid. Review the measures and take advantage of exclusion opportunities when applicable.

For our group, a lot of the measures that we chose, including the CQMs, are in a yes/no format. These types of measures are easier to capture in a structured format, which is the primary goal of Stage 1 Meaningful Use.

Regardless of where you end up, you need to be cognizant of the impact that these measures will have on your workflow. Some measures require new workflows to capture the data, while others can be automatically extracted from your certified EHR technology and no human intervention is required. The key here is to minimize burden on your patients, physicians, technologists, clerical staff, and administrative team.

Have you met with the meaningful use stakeholders at your organization? What can you tell us about that?

Goldszal: We realized early on that our MU Taskforce did not have to be as broad as we initially thought. In our practice, it boiled down to the RIS administrator, our legal counsel, a front desk supervisor, a chief technologist, and myself—the individuals that are most impacted by meaningful use.

Internal planning started with our bi-weekly steering committee. From that group we created a meaningful use working group that met on an ad-hoc basis for the first few months of planning our strategy. As we developed our strategy further and approached implementation, this group began to meet on a weekly basis. Much of the work at this stage involved preparing the training materials and working with our certified EHR technology vendor to test software and optimize new workflows.

Once we implemented our new workflows, this group became responsible for ongoing training and program maintenance. Preparing early and training your workforce at incremental steps will be instrumental to your success.

Have you met with your radiology IT vendors? What can you tell us about that?

Goldszal: We initially met with our RIS vendor in late 2010 to discuss meaningful use. At that point in time, their product was already certified for the program and had been since October 22, 2010. Let me also mention that while we technically call it a RIS, the technology that our vendor provides can be better described as an imaging EMR. The underlying technology offers much more than a traditional RIS and the benefits are seen in the newly supported workflows that are required for meaningful use.

Having access to complete certified EHR technology early on, and an IT partner that was very knowledgeable on the subject, made it easier for us to build our meaningful use strategy. Our vendor was ready with their software and was prepared to help us be ready too. Partnering with a radiology IT vendor that had meaningful use exposure proved valuable as we developed and executed our plan.

What have you and your organization done to plan your meaningful use technical and operational strategy?

Goldszal: We did a great deal of planning to ensure a smooth transition before, during, and after the implementation of our new workflows and processes. A clear communication plan was a key factor to our success as was being prepared with education and training materials. As I mentioned earlier, education and training falls under the responsibilities of our MU Taskforce. This core team has been instrumental in making sure that our radiologists, technologists, and office staff are educated and prepared to be successful with meaningful use today and into the future.

Does your organization plan to acquire and implement new technology to achieve meaningful use? If yes, what type of technology?

Goldszal: Fortunately, our imaging group did not have to acquire or implement new technology to comply with the program. We only needed to upgrade and test our existing technology to meet meaningful use requirements. Our RIS vendor was able to offer all of the necessary certified EHR technology that our practice needs to demonstrate and achieve Stage 1 Meaningful Use.

Do you have any comments about the online registration process with CMS?

Goldszal: Because the registration process is per EP, it was a bit long. Plan to set aside enough time to register each of your EPs and make sure you have all the required information at hand before starting the process. Having the prerequisites in place will help. With that said, it did take about thirty minutes on average to register a user. Sometimes it took longer, sometimes it took less. You need to pay attention to detail and plan for this. It's a little bit of a burden, but you have to do it.

What are your plans to monitor your imaging practice's meaningful use compliance?

Goldszal: Monitoring compliance is critical. You cannot just rely that this is working; you need to measure and track everything. You need to be quantitative here. And if you record it, you should be able to report it.

We have created dashboards to track numerators and denominators for individual EPs in real-time and graphically display if they fall above or below a specific threshold. Every week, our operating group runs a dashboard for each physician. If we find a problem, we take corrective action and immediately resolve the issue. You can only do this if you are measuring data on an ongoing basis and are able to take swift action. If you cannot adequately monitor your meaningful use compliance, it will be impossible to successfully attest.

Do you have any comments about the attestation process?

Goldszal: We just completed attestation and attention to detail is critical—just like it is for the registration process. Because the process is currently manual and requires page-by-page data entry for each EP, it takes fifteen to twenty minutes per radiologist. It is important not to rush the data entry and correctly pull the numbers for attestation. One word of advice is to set aside extra time. You will most likely need more than ninety-days in your first year to make post go-live corrections and adjustments. Again, begin early and avoid frustration by not waiting until the last minute to start.

Now that we've been through all that… what's next?

Goldszal: We will keep the momentum into next year and the focus on achieving meaningful use in Stages 2 and 3. We believe this is the beginning of a long journey and it's paramount to establish a solid foundation and a sustainable effort.

Any final thoughts or advice you would offer to other imaging providers that are developing their strategies for meaningful use? Any thoughts or hopes for future stages of the program?

Goldszal: Start early. If you haven't started yet, you really need to hustle. The key here is to be prepared and work with a certified technology provider that can support your strategy. You need to plan your work and work your plan.

Achieving meaningful use is doable, especially for radiology. We have developed, implemented, and adopted clinical information systems for more than twenty years and can conquer this challenge too. But, it needs to be an organized effort on the part of internal and external parties to be successful. If your radiology IT vendors are not ready, you will have difficult decisions to make.

You have to go through the growing pains. You must crawl and walk before you can run. And we are all in the crawling stage, which for this program means putting the data in a structured format. Once we do that, we can enable communication standards and begin to extract additional value out of this collective effort.

Some may believe that the cost of this program outweighs the benefits or that we are never going to get there. These are valid concerns, but if you take the positive out of it, there is no reason to believe that it's not the right direction to go. The program is evolving and our profession will evolve with it.

CHAPTER 14
A Conversation with Dr. David S. Mendelson

In this chapter, Dr. David S. Mendelson, Chief of Clinical Informatics and Director of Radiology, The Mount Sinai Medical Center, offers insight on learning the basics of the CMS EHR Incentive Programs, discusses meaningful use requirements and stakeholder meetings, reviews technical and operational strategies, and comments on the processes that surround meaningful use for radiologists.

About Dr. David S. Mendelson

David S. Mendelson, MD, FACR
Chief of Clinical Informatics, The Mount Sinai Medical Center
Director of Radiology Information Systems, The Mount Sinai Medical Center
Pulmonary Radiologist, The Mount Sinai Medical Center

David S. Mendelson has had a multi-faceted career in the domains of radiology and healthcare IT. He has served in several capacities at The Mount Sinai Medical Center.

In 1986, he was appointed the Director of Body CT-MRI in the Department of Radiology. While he was devoting the majority of his time to body imaging, he was also asked in 1990 to be the head of the DECRAD Radiology Information System (RIS). In 1992, his work led to his appointment as the Medical Director of Mount Sinai Clinical Information Services (TDS systems). In 1997, he was appointed as the Director of Radiology Information Systems. Subsequently, he expanded this interest and led the department's selection and implementation of a Picture Archiving and Communications System (PACS). Dr. Mendelson worked to develop a strategy to implement speech recognition and transcription software, which has exponentially shortened the time to report availability, and simultaneously saved several hundred thousand dollars a year.

In 2007, he was appointed as the Chief of Clinical Informatics for The Mount Sinai Medical Center, while still maintaining his teaching and diagnostic roles in chest imaging. His hands-on experience and knowledge of radiology informatics have led to leadership participation in the world of academic informatics. He currently serves on the Radiological Society of North America's (RSNA) Radiology Informatics Committee (RIC), where he is currently the Chairman of the Integrating the Healthcare Enterprise (IHE) subcommittee.

The activities described above have ultimately led to Dr. Mendelson's leadership in healthcare IT at a national and international level. He is the Co-Chair of the Board of Directors of Integrating the Healthcare Enterprise International (IHE), and much of his current activity is focused on image sharing and meaningful use.

A conversation on meaningful use

What have you and your organization done to educate yourselves on the fundamentals of meaningful use?

Mendelson: As soon as the ARRA of 2009 and HITECH Act were announced, our organization immediately established a cross-functional committee at the clinical level and began analyzing all of the relevant federal documents that were available at the time. We reviewed those documents line-by-line and distilled that information into a summary document that outlined things we had to do and questions we needed answered—it essentially became a working document to guide us.

As soon as the timelines were announced, we began planning on both the inpatient and ambulatory sides. We conducted a financial analysis that included billing data for Medicare and Medicaid and identified whom on the clinical staff, and later radiology staff, would be eligible for incentive opportunities.

Specific to radiology, we are staying apprised of the program by using resources like radiologyMU.org and medical society websites, speaking with colleagues about their strategies, and closely monitoring changes and clarifications to the regulations.

We really are focused on understanding the financial implications, who is eligible, who is not eligible, what our vendors are doing, and how they will support our strategy. We're also evaluating different approaches and looking at our RIS, our hospital EHR, as well as other certificated technology that we might be able to leverage to achieve meaningful use.

What steps have you taken to determine your eligibility and the financial impact of the CMS EHR Incentive Programs on your imaging practice?

Mendelson: We initially focused our attention on the clinical staff and later on our imaging practice. When determining eligibility, you need to take a look at both the Medicare and Medicaid versions of the program and their respective eligibility requirements. Like most imaging practices, our radiologists qualify as EPs under the Medicare version of the government program. We also had to consider the implications of practicing in a multi-site setting. Taking into account your eligibility and performing a multi-year cost analysis will provide justification for moving forward or delaying the program.

Have you determined your meaningful use measure requirements? If so, what did you discover during that process?

Mendelson: Early on in the process, I drew up a matrix and marked what we could exclude, what we definitely had to report, and those objectives and measures where it wasn't clear. I am always reviewing the matrix, updating it along the way, and sharing it with department management. This allows all levels in the department to become familiar with our position. It also gives them ideas of what might come so that they can better respond to changes in workflow and operations.

Have you met with the meaningful use stakeholders at your organization? What can you tell us about that?

Mendelson: Again, early on we put together a team with representation from across the board—including hospital IT staff, the office of the chief medical officer (both inpatient and ambulatory), our compliance officers, hospital operations, and faculty practice administration. We have routine meetings with all members, or a subset of members, as often as weekly to a more manageable monthly schedule—it all depends on how much is going on at the time with respect to meaningful use. Also, the work of this cross-functional group is reported to our strategic management team and the hospital CEO throughout the year.

Have you met with your radiology IT vendors? What can you tell us about that?

Mendelson: Yes, we have met with what we deem to be "key" radiology vendors for meaningful use. In the case of our organization, that's primarily our RIS vendor. We stay in touch with them through their formal user group meetings a couple times a year as well as through bi-weekly meetings where we discuss, among other topics, their meaningful use product road map and strategy.

What have you and your organization done to plan your meaningful use technical and operational strategy?

Mendelson: I think we share the same sentiment as other radiology practices in that there are a number of metrics that are not directly relevant to what a typical radiologist does on a daily basis. And to capture that information it will require workflow changes for the radiologists, workflow changes for the operations staff, and additional FTEs, which have the potential to diminish productivity across the board.

We have started to look at all of these things and are beginning to recognize the implications of potential changes, but we are waiting on the finalization of other projects before committing to any workflow changes. It's important to understand that each decision in the chain is linked. So until you know what products or technology you are going to introduce to demonstrate and achieve meaningful use, and how you are going to introduce them, you can't really go in-depth into the specifics of workflow changes.

Furthermore, you could debate exclusion opportunities for some of the program requirements. Recording vital signs is a good example. Many imaging practices may argue that you can exclude that particular measure, but in our ambulatory practice we do perform procedures in which blood pressure is occasionally taken. In this case, if you take a very literal interpretation of the law, as soon as you take one patient's blood pressure, you are required to do it for all patients.

The question then quickly becomes who is going to take the patient's blood pressure? Clerical staff? Nurses? Others? Or is the EP able to exclude that particular measure? Perhaps it only applies to some of our radiologists. You really need to analyze the final rules and evaluate each requirement for your imaging practice.

Does your organization plan to acquire and implement new technology to achieve meaningful use? If yes, what type of technology?

Mendelson: While we are still in the process of finalizing technology plans, we do have a few choices. One obvious choice is to leverage our hospital EMR and conduct meaningful use reporting through that system. We currently have an existing EMR interface, but we might extend that interface in order to meet program requirements and mine that data for each individual radiologist in our group. New workflows might include entering some data directly into the EMR to fill any gaps present with the RIS. The hospital IT department has expressed willingness to work with radiology to build those interfaces if that's the direction we decide to take.

The other option we are discussing is to implement a complete certified EHR that has been designed to accommodate radiology workflow. If we take that route, we envision having the certified EHR technology sit on top of our modular certified RIS. In this setup, the new technology would allow us to do as much work as possible in the existing RIS, cull the information into the overriding imaging EMR, and fill in the gaps. The key here is to explore all of your options and plan early.

Do you have any comments about the online registration process with CMS?

Mendelson: We have explored this already for our clinical staff, but not yet for our radiologists. Currently, there is no batch registration, but at least CMS allows authorized third parties to register on behalf of the EP. Even so, the third party that is registering each EP is required to obtain a few pieces of information and getting that initial data can be challenging. We have heard stories that some individuals are able to obtain the necessary data quickly, while it has taken others significantly more time to do so. All in all, if you have all of the information that is needed, the registration process is fairly streamlined, but it still requires each EP to be registered individually.

What are your plans to monitor your imaging practice's meaningful use compliance?

Mendelson: We already produce monthly report cards for each of our clinicians and plan to replicate the process when we demonstrate meaningful use in our radiology practice. Once we establish our final exclusions and reporting requirements, we plan to leverage the experience with our clinical staff, but acknowledge this will require significant tweaks for our radiology EPs.

14

Do you have any comments about the attestation process?

Mendelson: A subset of our cross-functional team is responsible for the attestation process, which falls under the auspices of our CMOs. That's why the CMOs were directly involved from the start.

Now that we've been through all that... what's next?

Mendelson: Our current intent is to collect maximum EP incentives starting in 2012. However, final determination will depend upon the value of the incentive opportunity, factoring in implementation costs and workflow changes, to make sure that the net gain is worthwhile given the current economic environment in radiology. Even if the gain is less than we had hoped for, we plan to demonstrate meaningful use well before the penalties kick in.

Any final thoughts or advice you would offer to other imaging providers that are developing their strategies for meaningful use? Any thoughts or hopes for future stages of the program?

Mendelson: If you have any belief that you are going to be involved with these programs, you need to have at least one point person from attending staff and one from finance actively engaged and monitoring program changes. It's a dynamic topic and you can't learn it overnight. You really need to review all available material, look at everything you have to do, and stay on top of program requirements. Bottom line is not to be naïve about it.

While the radiology community acknowledges the public health benefits of the programs, with respect to current and future stages, there are better ways to improve the quality of care by radiologists and the imaging profession in general. There should really be meaningful use measures that are specific to medical specialties. To provide a "real" contribution to medical workflow, future stages of the program should provision such efforts as clinical decision support to ensure appropriate imaging, encourage image sharing to reduce unnecessary exams, and promote the tracking and monitoring of radiation dosing. While there might be difficulties with implementing all of this, it's well worth the effort.

Part III:
IMAGING PROVIDER PERSPECTIVES

CHAPTER 15
A Conversation with Steven F. Fischer

In this chapter, Steven F. Fischer, CIO, Center for Diagnostic Imaging, offers insight on learning the basics of the CMS EHR Incentive Programs, discusses meaningful use requirements and stakeholder meetings, reviews technical and operational strategies, and comments on the processes that surround meaningful use for radiologists.

About Steven F. Fischer

Steven F. Fischer
Chief Information Officer, Center for Diagnostic Imaging

With more than thirty years of experience in software development, and seventeen years in health care, Steven F. Fischer, Chief Information Officer at the Center for Diagnostic Imaging (CDI), is responsible for the strategic and tactical aspects of CDI's business and clinical systems and infrastructure. This responsibility extends to operational support, including business process and training, as well as biomedical engineering, and transcription.

A conversation on meaningful use

What have you and your organization done to educate yourselves on the fundamentals of meaningful use?

Fischer: The most valuable information came directly from CMS—including details about incentive payouts, eligibility determination, and general guidance and clarification. We also reviewed the regulations, certification processes and test scripts, and looked at trade magazines as well as a variety of online resources. We basically scoured all of the available content to find whatever information we could.

What steps have you taken to determine your eligibility and the financial impact of the CMS EHR Incentive Programs on your imaging practice?

Fischer: Initially, we worked with our CFO and pulled together information relevant to eligibility and financials. We asked ourselves:

- Are our radiologists eligible?

- Do they meet the thresholds of the program?

- Is radiologist participation realistic?

- What are the potential dollars available?

- Do we believe we can meet and demonstrate all of the requirements of Stage 1 Meaningful Use?

Our practice was also involved in lobbying efforts for the radiology community before Stage 1 Meaningful Use requirements were finalized. As a result of all of this, we felt comfortable that we could qualify and meet the initial round of requirements.

Have you determined your meaningful use measure requirements? If so, what did you discover during that process?

Fischer: Yes, we have determined our specific requirements. Initially, we looked at all of them and further determined measure requirements for each individual radiologist. Since our radiologists are subspecialized, and the reporting requirements vary based on practice type classification, we needed to take that into account. We came to the conclusion that there were differences between our diagnostic radiologists and interventional radiologists and that the metrics for those two classes of eligible professionals are different.

Have you met with the meaningful use stakeholders at your organization? What can you tell us about that?

Fischer: Given the structure of our organization, our primary stakeholders are our radiology partners, whom we meet with on a quarterly basis. Early on, we educated them on the topic of meaningful use and reached general business agreement that this is something that our radiologists wanted to move forward with. We discussed the logistics of how the program would be funded, how the incentives would be allocated, and how to put the necessary systems in place to meet the requirements.

Once the decision was made to move forward, we built our meaningful use project team. These individuals meet weekly with status updates and review where we are in the process, discuss updates on change management and training, examine implementation requirements, and prepare for any changes with the front desk, technologist, and radiologist workflow.

Have you met with your radiology IT vendors?
What can you tell us about that?

Fischer: Early on, we talked to our RIS vendor. That was really the only vendor we needed to have discussions with as their product is very encompassing and already possesses much of the functionality of an EMR. We approached our RIS vendor about their meaningful use plans and discussed how they would support our business and strategy. We were comfortable with the solution they provided and were given the components needed to integrate into our existing product to meet program requirements.

What have you and your organization done to plan your meaningful use technical and operational strategy?

Fischer: First, we met with our radiologists and identified the metrics that we need to report to CMS. After that, we reviewed each measure and determined which ones would require us to attach additional information or change our existing processes in order to capture the information.

Some measures, such as the patient's preferred language and BMI, are not calculated and reported as part of our existing workflow. Our team examined all of the measures and met with operational personnel, including front desk staff and supervisors. We discussed how the information would best be captured within the constraints that we have to operate within.

In terms of operational strategy, we initially began educating our associates in late 2010. Starting with change management first, we explained meaningful use and got our staff familiar and comfortable with what's coming. This operational review also included putting together design specifications to make sure that our support teams and radiology EPs would be comfortable with any potential workflow changes.

Does your organization plan to acquire and implement new technology to achieve meaningful use? If yes, what type of technology?

Fischer: We plan to leverage our existing RIS. However, in order to demonstrate meaningful use, we needed to implement additional functionality from our RIS vendor to extend the current offering so that we can meet our meaningful use objectives and measures.

Do you have any comments about the online registration process with CMS?

Fischer: We just began the process in terms of registration. From our early experience, it is relatively straightforward. The ability to assign authorized third parties will make the process even easier to complete.

What are your plans to monitor your imaging practice's meaningful use compliance?

Fischer: We already have an extensive data warehouse and business intelligence capability in place today. As a result, we are in the process of expanding that technology to include additional meaningful use data elements. Once we have everything in place, we plan to build individual provider reports and EP dashboards to deliver program compliance and incentive payment status to each radiologist moving forward.

Do you have any comments about the attestation process?

Fischer: First off, we don't know what we don't know yet. While attestation is a manual process today, the promise is that this will be automated with electronic attestation in the future. However, there are currently no formal specifications as to what the electronic attestation format will be and how data will be submitted. We have not yet reached this stage, but anticipate a positive experience as a result of properly preparing for the attestation process.

Now that we've been through all that… what's next?

Fischer: We plan to begin demonstrating meaningful use in the first half of 2012.

Any final thoughts or advice you would offer to other imaging providers that are developing their strategies for meaningful use? Any thoughts or hopes for future stages of the program?

Fischer: To be successful, it's better to get started sooner than later. You need to decide exactly what you are going to do and how you are going to get there. As for future stages, it would be really nice to see an increased focus on technology and processes that are more representative of the roles and responsibilities of medical specialists. Technology, such as decision support for diagnostic image ordering appropriateness, will have a greater impact on radiologists, while also improving the overall patient care workflow.

Part IV:
RESOURCES AND STAYING INFORMED

In this final section, we review ongoing advocacy efforts and information related to evolution of the regulations, offer additional resources and tools, recap Stage 1 Meaningful Use, and briefly look at what the future might hold for the CMS EHR Incentive Programs.

CHAPTER 16
Advocacy Efforts

Stay up-to-date on advocacy efforts.

To stay on top of medical imaging society advocacy efforts that are underway, learn about how you can help, and to stay informed on how radiology EPs are being represented at the federal level, scan the QR code above or go to **advocacy.theMUguide.com.**

In this chapter, we take a brief look at the countless advocacy efforts initiated by medical imaging societies since the early days of these government programs. We also discuss ongoing efforts that will ensure better representation for radiology professionals in future stages of meaningful use.

Meaningful use advocacy efforts

Since the passing of the ARRA in 2009, a number of medical imaging societies and organizations have worked together to lobby the ONC and CMS and ensure better representation with respect to meaningful use for radiologists. The ACR has been, and continues to be, responsible for driving many of these efforts. Through the combined efforts of the ACR Government Relations Department, ACR IT and Informatics Committee, and Government Relations Subcommittee, they have had, and continue to have, a significant impact on meaningful use on behalf of the nation's practicing radiologists.

The primary goals of the ACR, with respect to meaningful use, include but are not limited to:

• Promoting specification of measures and exclusions for radiologists.

• Urging for the removal of the ONC requirements for possession of all certification criteria.

• Expanding the definition of radiology results to include images—promoting image sharing and distribution via EHR technology.

• Promoting the use of ACR Appropriateness Criteria® (AC) for imaging clinical decision support (CDS)—participating in the CMS CDS Demonstration Project and testifying for the use of ACR AC in meaningful use measures.

ACR timeline of MU initiatives and public comments

Since May 2009, the ACR has participated in more than sixty ONC meetings and teleconferences related to the topic of meaningful use. In June 2009, the ACR commented to the ONC on the draft meaningful use matrix, shaping the initial set of recommendations to address concerns within the radiology community. Shortly thereafter, the ACR published a detailed meaningful use FAQ webpage that it still maintains for the imaging community today. By October 2009, the ACR had held meetings with ONC staff and submitted testimony on meaningful use for radiologists.

A few months later, in January 2010, the ACR provided analysis of the CMS Notice of Proposed Rulemaking and ONC Interim Final Rule. Two months later, the ACR, with the ABR, RSNA, and SIIM, provided joint comments to CMS and the ONC. In April 2010, the ACR worked with the RSNA RadLex Chair to comment to the ONC Vocabulary Task Force. In July 2010, one year after launching their online FAQ, the ACR drafted a summary document and updated FAQ based on the final meaningful use rules. Toward the end of 2010, the ACR, along with Pathologists and Anesthesiologists, drafted a letter to the ONC. It was at this time that they also commented on Stage 2 Meaningful Use clinical quality measure concepts.

Their efforts continued through 2011. In January 2011, the ACR, joined by the RSNA, commented on the ONC RFI regarding the PCAST report. One month later, they commented on draft Stage 2 Meaningful Use measure recommendations. One month after that, in March 2011, the ACR verbally commented to the full HITPC and ONC MU Workgroup. Following the verbal comments in March 2011, the ACR testified to the ONC MU Workgroup on specialty care, imaging, and CDS.

Representation for medical specialists

A pivotal event for advocacy took place on May 13, 2011. Representatives from five medical specialties, including radiology, met with the Meaningful Use Workgroup of the ONC in Washington, DC and offered suggestions for Stage 2 guidelines. Members of the ACR IT and Informatics Committee represented the radiology community and presented strong arguments, citing specific examples as to how specialists, such as those in the medical imaging field, could contribute to health care coordination, efficiency, and quality improvements that will improve the specialty care of patients.

In June 2011, the ONC MU Workgroup stated they would submit a separate recommendation for specialists later in the year. During the same month, CMS released a clarification about the definition of "seen by the EP."

In early October 2011, a series of meetings took place to further advance specialist involvement in the program—including a meeting with the ONC HIT Policy Committee Meaningful Use Workgroup to discuss experiences and potential Stage 3 Meaningful Use concepts, a meeting with the National Coordinator for HIT to discuss improving program requirements, and a discussion with the ONC HIT Policy Committee Meaningful Use Workgroup (Specialist Subgroup) about meaningful use gaps and opportunities regarding specialists.

It's clear that the ACR, and other medical societies, are acting in the best interest of their members and the specialist community at large. With ongoing involvement from the ACR's government relations arm and others, the radiology community will continue to have a strong voice on meaningful use.

16

16

CHAPTER 17
Resources and Important Dates

Take advantage of available resources.

To view the most recent list of resources and contact details made available by the federal government as well as important program dates, scan the QR code above or go to **resources.theMUguide.com.**

In this chapter, we take a look at additional resource opportunities to help you on the road to meaningful use and outline a few important dates related to the program.

Health Information Technology Extension Program (HITEP)

Section 3012 (Health Information Technology Implementation Assistance) of the HITECH Act provides supportive services for the Health Information Technology Extension Program. This program awarded cooperative agreements for the establishment of Regional Extension Centers (RECs) that offer technical assistance, guidance, and information on best practices to support and accelerate health care providers' efforts to become meaningful users. The program also established a national Health Information Technology Research Center (HITRC) to serve as a resource for regional centers.

Health Information Technology Research Center (HITRC)

The Health Information Technology Research Center (HITRC) is a separately funded initiative under the HIT Extension Program. The purpose of the HITRC is to gather relevant information on effective practices from a wide variety of sources across the country and help the Regional Extension Centers collaborate with one another on relevant stakeholders to identify and share best practices in EHR adoption, effective use, and provider support. This group will build a virtual community of shared learning to advance best practices that support providers' adoption and meaningful use of EHRs.

Regional Extension Centers (RECs)

Regional Extension Centers (RECs) were created in 2009 under the HITECH Act and finalized in September 2010. Under the HITECH Act, $677 million is allocated through 2012 to support the nationwide system of 62 RECs. RECs will help physicians, clinics, and hospitals to move from paper-based medical records to EHRs. These organizations target their assistance to eligible primary care providers in smaller practices as well as small and rural hospitals and public health clinics. They also serve as resources for all providers in a given geographic region.

2010–2012 Regional Extension Centers

The following is the complete list of RECs that was finalized in September 2010. The performance of each REC will be evaluated every two years to determine if continued federal support for the center is in the best interest of the extension program.

List of Regional Extension Centers

Alabama (AL)
Alabama Regional Extension Center
http://www.al-rec.org

Alaska (AK)
Alaska eHealth Network
http://www.ak-ehealth.com

Arkansas (AR)
HIT Arkansas
http://www.hitarkansas.com

Arizona (AZ)
Arizona Health-e Connection (AzHeC)
http://www.azhec.org

California (CA)
CalHIPSO (North)
CalHIPSO (South)
http://www.calhipso.org

CalOptima Foundation
http://www.caloptima.org

HITEC-LA
http://www.hitec-la.org

Colorado (CO)
Colorado Regional Extension Center (CORHIO)
http://www.corhio.org

Connecticut (CT)
eHealth Connecticut
http://www.ehealthconnecticut.org

District of Columbia (DC)
eHealth DC
http://www.ehealthdc.org

National Indian Health Board (NIHB)
http://www.nihb.org

Delaware (DE)
Quality Insights of Delaware
http://www.qide.org/de

Florida (FL)
Rural and North Florida Regional Extension Center
http://www.chcalliance.org/Services/RegionalExtensionCenter.aspx

South Florida Regional Extension Center Collaborative
http://www.southfloridarec.org

Central Florida REC
http://www.ucf-rec.org

PaperFree Florida
http://health.usf.edu/paperfree/index.htm

Georgia (GA)
Georgia HITREC
http://www.ga-hitrec.org

Hawaii (HI)
Hawaii-Pacific REC
http://www.hawaiihie.org

Iowa (IA)
Health Information Technology Regional Extension Center (Iowa HITREC)
http://www.telligenhitrec.org

Idaho (ID)
See Washington (WA)

Illinois (IL)
Illinois Health Information Technology Regional Extension Center (IL-HITREC)
http://www.ilhitrec.org

Chicago Health Information Technology Regional
Extension Center (CHITREC)
http://www.chitrec.org

Indiana (IN)
Purdue University
http://www.ihitec.purdue.edu

Kansas (KS)
Kansas Foundation for Medical Care, Inc. (KFMC)
http://www.kfmc.org/rec

Kentucky (KY)
University of Kentucky Research Foundation
http://www.ky-rec.org

Louisiana (LA)
Louisiana Health Care Quality Forum
http://www.lhcqf.org

Massachusetts (MA)
Massachusetts Technology Park Corporation
http://www.maehi.org/rec

Maryland (MD)
Chesapeake Regional Information System for Our Patients
http://www.crisphealth.org

Maine (ME)
HealthInfoNet
http://www.hinfonet.org

Michigan (MI)
Michigan Center for Effective IT Adoption (M-CEITA)
http://www.mceita.org

Minnesota (MN) and North Dakota (ND)
Regional Extension Assistance Center for
Health Information Technology (REACH)
http://www.khareach.org

Missouri (MO)
Missouri HIT Assistance Center
http://www.assistancecenter.missouri.edu

Mississippi (MS)
Mississippi Regional Extension Center
http://www.eqhealthsolutions.com

Montana (MT) and Wyoming (WY)
Mountain Pacific Quality Health Foundation (MPQHF)
http://www.mpqhf.org

North Carolina (NC)
University of North Carolina AHEC REC
http://www.med.unc.edu/ahec

North Dakota (ND)
See Minnesota (MN)

Nebraska (NE)
Wide River Technology Extension Center
http://www.widerivertec.org

New Hampshire (NH)
Regional Extension Center of New Hampshire
http://www.maehc.org

New Jersey (NJ)
New Jersey Institute of Technology
http://www.njhitec.org

New Mexico (NM)
Lovelace Clinic Foundation - LCF Research
http://www.lcfresearch.org

Nevada (NV)
See Utah (UT)

New York (NY)
NYC REACH
http://www.nycreach.org

New York eHealth Collaborative (NYeC)
http://www.nyehealth.org

Ohio (OH)
HealthBridge Tri-State REC (for select areas in Ohio, Indiana & Kentucky)
http://www.healthbridge.org

Ohio Health Information Partnership (OHIP)
http://www.ohiponline.org

Oklahoma (OK)
Oklahoma Foundation for Medical Quality (OFMQ)
http://www.ofmq.com

Oregon (OR)
Oregon's Health Information Technology Extension Center (O-HITECH)
http://o-hitec.org

Pennsylvania (PA)
Quality Insights of Pennsylvania (Eastern)
Quality Insights of Pennsylvania (Western)
http://www.qipa.org/pa

Puerto Rico (PR)
Ponce School of Medicine
http://www.psm.edu

Rhode Island (RI)
Rhode Island Quality Institute
http://www.riqi.org

South Carolina (SC)
Center for Information Technology Implementation
Assistance in South Carolina (CITIA-SC)
http://www.healthsciencessc.org

South Dakota (SD)
healthPOINT
http://www.healthpoint.dsu.edu

Tennessee (TN)
Qsource
http://www.tnrec.org

Texas (TX)
North Texas Regional Extension Center
http://www.ntrec.org

West Texas Health Information Technology
Regional Extension Center (WT-HITREC)
http://www.wtxhitrec.org

CentrEast Regional Extension Center
http://centreastrec.org

Gulf Coast Regional Extension Center
http://www.uthouston.edu/gcrec

Utah (UT) and Nevada (NV)
HealthInsight
http://www.healthinsight.org

Virginia (VA)
Virginia Health Quality Center (VHQC)
http://www.vhqc.org

Vermont (VT)
Vermont Information Technology Leaders
http://www.vitl.net

Washington (WA) and Idaho (ID)
Washington-Idaho Regional Extension Center (WIREC)
http://www.wirecqh.org

Wisconsin (WI)
Wisconsin Health Information Technology Extension Center
http://www.whitec.org

West Virginia (WV)
West Virginia Health Improvement Institute
http://www.wvhealthimprovement.org

Wyoming (WY)
See Montana (MT)

CMS EHR Incentive Programs Listserv

Another great resource is the CMS EHR Incentive Programs Listserv, which offers timely, authoritative information about the government program. Through this system, CMS keeps EPs informed about upcoming deadlines, answers questions and addresses concerns about the program, circulates updates, and notifies subscribers of new FAQ documents related to the incentive programs. To subscribe to the CMS EHR Incentive Programs Listserv, go to **ehrlistserv.theMUguide.com.**

Important program dates for radiologists

There are many important program dates, but the following are key program dates for eligible professionals participating in the Medicare version of the CMS EHR Incentive Programs.

January 1, 2011: Reporting year begins for eligible professionals.

January 3, 2011: Registration for the Medicare EHR Incentive Program begins.

April 2011: Attestation for the Medicare EHR Incentive Program begins.

May 2011: EHR Incentive Payments begin.

October 3, 2011: Last day for eligible professionals to begin their ninety-day reporting period for calendar year 2011 for the Medicare EHR Incentive Program.

December 31, 2011: Reporting year ends for eligible professionals.

February 29, 2012: Last day for EPs to register and attest to receive an EHR Incentive Payment for calendar year 2011.

June 2012: Stage 2 Meaningful Use Final Rule to be issued.

2013-2014: Stage 2 Meaningful Use begins.

2015: Stage 3 Meaningful Use begins. Medicare payment adjustments begin for EPs who are not demonstrating meaningful use.

2016: Last year to receive an EHR Incentive Payment.

Stay Up-to-Date: As resources and links have a tendency to change frequently, we encourage you to visit the companion website to this guide for a current list of RECs and important program dates. For an up-to-date list, scan the QR code at the beginning of this chapter or go to **resources.theMUguide.com.**

17

CHAPTER 18
Beyond Stage 1, Preparing for Stages 2 and 3

Stay up-to-date on Stages 2 and 3.

With Stages 2 and 3 Meaningful Use around the corner, program regulations are taking shape, but still changing on an ongoing basis. To learn about program changes and updates, scan the QR code above or go to **beyondstage1.theMUguide.com**.

In this chapter, we take a look at the direction the program is taking and what might come in future stages of meaningful use.

The future of meaningful use

The requirements for Stage 1 Meaningful Use have been established and its set of well-defined objectives will undoubtedly act as the foundation for subsequent stages of the CMS EHR Incentive Programs. Since the time that the Final Rule was released in July 2010, health care professionals have been tackling existing regulations in anticipation of future program requirements that expand on this foundation by promoting quality, structured information exchange, safety, efficiency, and population health improvements.

With Stage 2 now slated for 2014, and Stage 3 for 2015, things are moving rapidly. The next step in the meaningful use process expands on Stage 1 by focusing on a greater level of engagement and communication with patients. In the Stage 2 Proposed Rule, nearly all Stage 1 core and menu set objectives have been retained, but some have been eliminated, replaced, or combined. Moreover, there are proposed changes to Stage 1 criteria as well as new Stage 2 objectives that have greater applicability to specialists.

In general, the Stage 2 Proposed Rule:

• Increases flexibility and reduces burden on providers and vendors.

• Emphasizes patient engagement, access to information, and HIE.

• Promotes greater usability and encryption requirements.

Proposed Stage 2 objectives that have more applicability to medical specialists, include:

• Imaging results and information accessible through certified EHR technology.

• Capability to identify and report cancer cases to a State cancer registry, except where prohibited, and in accordance with applicable law and practice.

• Capability to identify and report specific cases to a specialized registry (other than a cancer registry), except where prohibited, and in accordance with applicable law and practice.

Along with provider requirements, the definition of certified EHR technology continues to evolve. For instance, the proposed revision to the Standards, Implementation Specifications, and Certification Criteria and Permanent Certification Program focuses on flexibility, clearer requirements, increased interoperability, and the use of standards. Despite this guidance, it is important to remember that details can, and will, change before the Stage 2 Final Rules are issued by CMS and ONC. For the latest information about the next stage of meaningful use, go to **beyondstage1.theMUguide.com**.

With Stage 3 Meaningful Use on the heels of Stage 2, the focus will be on promoting improvements in quality, safety, and efficiency—decision support for high-priority conditions, patient access to self-management tools, access to comprehensive patient data, and improving the overall population health.

CMS will ultimately determine how aggressive future stages of meaningful use will be and the specifics surrounding the objectives and measures. Fortunately for radiologists, the advocacy efforts of major medical imaging societies—including the ACR, RSNA, ABR, SIIM, and others—are well underway and the inclusion of radiology-specific recommendations in the Stage 2 Proposed Rules are a testament to those efforts. These specialty societies are working aggressively with federal agencies to encourage better representation for medical specialists in future program regulations. Specific to medical imaging, recommendations for improving medical imaging care include providing meaningful use functionality and measures for structured reporting, critical findings communication, access to key image data, and recording and monitoring radiation dose.

Ongoing education is key

The federal regulations surrounding future stages of the CMS EHR Incentive Programs are in a constant state of flux. With these rapid changes in health care reform, continually educating yourself on meaningful use initiatives and staying informed of the ever-changing regulations will be instrumental to achieving a successful implementation and demonstration of meaningful use at your organization.

18

CHAPTER 19
Frequently Asked Questions for Radiologists

Read the most current FAQs online.

As with any government program that changes over time, so do the frequently asked questions. To view the most current list of FAQs that are relevant to radiology EPs, scan the QR code above or go to **faqs.theMUguide.com.**

In this chapter, we address some of the most commonly asked questions about meaningful use and radiology professionals—discussing general FAQs, eligibility and participation, incentives and penalties, objectives and measures, product certification, and registration and attestation.

General FAQs

What is "meaningful use"?

Meaningful use is synonymous with the CMS EHR Incentive Programs. It includes the Medicare and Medicaid EHR Incentive Programs for eligible professionals (EPs) and eligible hospitals (EHs) under the American Recovery and Reinvestment Act of 2009. The program is designed to encourage health care providers to use certified electronic health record (EHR) technology and demonstrate compliance through a series of measures and criteria.

Are there any special program considerations for radiologists participating in the CMS EHR Incentive Programs?

No, the government program was designed as one-size-fits-all and does not provide special considerations for specialty physicians such as radiologists. However, EPs are encouraged to take advantage of exclusion opportunities if they meet the circumstances of the exclusion. Selecting the best fit measures will alleviate some of the program reporting requirements. If an EP is unable to meet all non-excludable measures, then the EP would not be eligible to receive incentive payments under rules of the program.

Where do I go for more information?

In addition to online resources like radiologyMU.org and government program websites, an imaging practice or EP may choose to contact a Regional Extension Center (REC) in their area (see chapter 17 for a complete list of RECs and contact information for the center in your region). These regional non-profit organizations, partially funded by the federal government, provide EHR consulting services to EPs. Primary care and rural health care providers are given priority, but they also serve as information centers for radiology EPs and other specialists.

Eligibility and participation

19

If a radiology EP is under the practice meaningful use program, can he/she participate in the hospital program?

Most hospitals will be applying as an eligible hospital (EH), not eligible professional (EP), under the program. Most radiologists qualify as EPs. Some hospitals have undertaken the effort of acquiring the technology necessary for both programs (typically a hospital with a large number of closely affiliated physicians). Your group will need to check with the hospitals that your radiology EPs service to see if they are applying for either, or both, programs. If so, it will be the radiology EP's choice to participate or not in the hospital's program.

If the hospital is participating in their own meaningful use program, will any of the incentive payments received by the hospital be passed on to the non-employed radiology EP?

Even if the radiology EP works exclusively in a hospital setting (assuming they qualify for the program by reading less than 90 percent inpatient and ER), the imaging group could still manage the EP compliance and attestation. The ease of this approach will vary based on how much of the technology the imaging practice supplies to these hospitals (mainly the RIS, but also the reporting solution and potentially the PACS). If this technology were owned by the hospital(s) there would need to be interfaces to extract the required measures needed for monitoring and attestation. Also, the "seen by the EP" clarification posted on the CMS FAQ website states that all meaningful use measures that use the phrase may be defined by the EP consistently across their practice to exclude much, but not all, of their practice activity from the program. That means you could possibly opt to exclude hospital activity from radiology EP compliance. Therefore, even if it represented a majority, but not all, of the EP's practice activity, it could be excluded, allowing your imaging practice to measure minimal activity performed in the practice and still allow the EP to theoretically comply.

Incentives and penalties

Which geographic areas qualify for incentive payments?

According to the ARRA and HITECH Act, eligible providers in all fifty U.S. states, the District of Columbia, Puerto Rico, the U.S. Virgin Islands, Guam, American Samoa, and the Northern Mariana Islands qualify for the incentive programs.

What is the maximum total incentive payment that an EP can receive under the Medicare EHR Incentive Program?

An EP that successfully demonstrates meaningful use by 2012 can receive up to $44,000 over the life of the incentive program. The total incentive opportunity goes down for each year that passes before an EP first successfully demonstrates and attests to meaningful use. After 2015, penalties in the form of payment reductions kick in if an EP does not demonstrate meaningful use.

Under the Medicare EHR Incentive Program, what is the earliest date that payment adjustments will kick in?

For Medicare EPs that do not demonstrate meaningful use of certified EHR technology, payment adjustments will begin in 2015.

As a radiology EP, how do I receive a Medicare EHR Incentive Payment?

In order for an EP to receive incentive payments under the Medicare version of the program, they will need to (1) successfully register for the program on the CMS program website (2) meet meaningful use criteria using certified EHR technology (3) demonstrate meaningful use by successfully attesting that they have met program criteria using certified EHR technology.

If a radiology EP provides service exclusively in a hospital setting, does he or she qualify for meaningful use incentive payments?

Each radiology EP is eligible to receive incentive payments from only one program, so in this case the radiology EP can participate in either program, but not both. That said, many hospitals that are creating an EP solution for their affiliated physicians will most likely be asking for a portion of the incentives from the EPs since the hospital is paying for the cost of the technology and attestation solutions.

How long does it take to receive a payment check?

Once an EP has successfully demonstrated meaningful use and attested using the Medicare and Medicaid EHR Incentive Programs Registration and Attestation System, incentive payments will be made within eight weeks. Note that CMS will hold payments until an EP meets the annual billable threshold.

How are incentive payments made?

Payments are made to the TIN number that an EP chooses during program registration—either the individual EP or the imaging practice. An EP's first payment will be made by electronic funds transfer or paper check depending how the EP currently receives payment.

Objectives and measures

I am a radiology EP that provides care in a group practice. Does each provider need to demonstrate meaningful use or can it be achieved by averaging data at the group level?

Incentive program payments are based on each EP, not an entire practice. Each radiology EP in your imaging group is required to demonstrate meaningful use by reporting and attesting to individual measures. The CMS Final Rule declined the adoption of an alternative means to demonstrate meaningful use through group level data aggregation.

How many measures do I need to report for Stage 1 Meaningful Use?

As a radiology EP participating in the Medicare EHR Incentive Program, you will need to report on 15 core set measures, up to five out of 10 menu set measures, and six clinical quality measures (three core/alternate core and three discretionary) unless exclusion criteria is met. See chapter 8 for details about exclusion opportunities based on typical radiologist practice types.

Is it true that I need to "possess" certified EHR technology even if I can claim exclusion for specific measures?

Yes, the regulations currently require all participants in the incentive program to "possess" EHR technology that is tested and certified for all 33 Certification Criteria. The ONC considers "possession" of certified EHR technology to be either the physical possession of a medium on which a certified Complete EHR or combination of certified EHR modules resides, or a legally enforceable right by an eligible provider to access and use, at its discretion, the capabilities of the certified technology.

If certified EHR technology possessed by an EP includes the ability to choose CQMs from the discretionary set that are not indicated by the EHR developer or on the Certified Health Information Technology Product List as tested and certified by an ONC-ATCB, can the EP submit the results of those CQMs to CMS as part of their meaningful use attestation?

Yes, the EP can submit results for CQMs in the discretionary set calculated by certified EHR technology, even if those CQMs were not individually tested and certified by an ONC-ATCB. CMS expects to revisit the requirements in more detail for later stages of meaningful use as well as the corresponding certification requirements.

Product certification

Does my EHR technology have to be certified prior to beginning the EHR reporting period?

No, you may begin to demonstrate meaningful use prior to product certification, but certification must be obtained prior to the end of the EHR reporting period. If you begin the EHR reporting period prior to your vendor's obtaining product certification, be aware that you are at risk for disqualification if the EHR technology you are using requires any changes for certification.

If my radiology IT vendor is not going to certify their product, can our practice get it certified for meaningful use?

Yes, however, most vendors will submit for Modular or Complete EHR certification on behalf of their customers. If your imaging practice has developed technology that you use, you may consider obtaining certification if the technology will be used as part of your meaningful use strategy.

Does it matter which ONC-ATCB certifies our vendor's technology? Is one better than another?

No, all ONC-ATCBs must comply with the certification regulations published by the ONC. Therefore, it is not important which certifying body has approved your IT vendor's solution for compliance with meaningful use, but rather which components the technology is certified for.

Registration and attestation

19

When and where can I register for the Medicare EHR Incentive Program?

Now. As of January 3, 2011, registration for the Medicare EHR Incentive Program went live. An EP may register anytime up until they are ready to attest. Registration is conducted through the Medicare and Medicaid EHR Incentive Programs Registration and Attestation System, which can be found on the CMS EHR Incentive Programs website at **ehrincentiveprograms.theMUguide.com.**

What is the EP reporting period?

The Medicare EP reporting period for the first year is ninety consecutive days within the calendar year. For subsequent years of participation, the reporting period is the entire calendar year.

Is there anything I can do to prepare for attestation?

Yes, CMS has developed a Meaningful Use Attestation Calculator that allows a provider to test whether he or she would successfully demonstrate meaningful use for the CMS EHR Incentive Programs. The calculator can be found on the incentive program website at **ehrincentiveprograms. theMUguide.com.**

How do I calculate my numbers if I am a radiology EP that practices in multiple practice settings?

For radiology EPs who practice in both inpatient and outpatient settings (e.g. a hospital and an imaging center), and where certified EHR technology is available at both, the EP should base both the numerators and denominators for meaningful use objectives on the number of unique patients at the imaging center, since this is where they are eligible to receive payments from the Medicare EHR Incentive Program.

How long do we need to keep our meaningful use records?

While you should store this information in a persistent database, CMS requires that documentation be kept for a minimum of six years. At any point, CMS may audit your imaging practice and you may be required to have this documentation available.

CHAPTER 20
Acronyms

View the most current list of meaningful use acronyms online.

While the list of acronyms used throughout meaningful use documentation and literature is fairly static, new acronyms are bound to arise. To view a complete list of program-related acronyms, scan the QR code above or go to **acronyms.theMUguide.com.**

With more than one thousand pages of regulations, the CMS EHR Incentive Programs documentation has introduced dozens of new acronyms. While not fully comprehensive, the list below outlines the common acronyms used throughout this guide and meaningful use literature.

ANSI American National Standards Institute
A private non-profit organization that oversees the development of voluntary consensus standards for products, services, processes, systems, and personnel in the United States.

ARRA American Recovery and Reinvestment Act of 2009
Commonly referred to as "the Stimulus" or "The Recovery Act," ARRA is an economic stimulus package enacted by the 111th United States Congress in February 2009 and signed into law on February 17, 2009, by President Barack Obama.

CAH Critical Access Hospital
Hospitals that are certified to receive cost-based reimbursement from Medicare. The reimbursement that CAHs receive is intended to improve their financial performance and thereby reduce hospital closures.

CCR Continuity of Care Record
A patient health summary standard developed jointly by ASTM International, the Massachusetts Medical Society (MMS), the Healthcare Information and Management Systems Society (HIMSS), the American Academy of Family Physicians (AAFP), the American Academy of Pediatrics (AAP), and other health informatics vendors.

CDA Clinical Document Architecture
An XML-based markup standard intended to specify the encoding, structure, and semantics of clinical documents for exchange.

CDC Centers for Disease Control and Prevention
The United States federal agency under the Department of Health and Human Services that works to protect public health and safety by providing information to enhance health decisions and promote health through partnerships with state departments and other organizations.

CFR Code of Federal Regulations
The codification of the general and permanent rules and regulations published in the Federal Register by the executive departments and agencies of the United States Federal Government.

CHPL Certified Health IT Product List
The authoritative and comprehensive listing of Complete EHRs and EHR Modules that have been tested and certified for meaningful use.

CMS Centers for Medicare & Medicaid Services
The federal agency within HHS that administers the Medicare program and works in partnership with state governments to administer Medicaid, the State Children's Health Insurance Program (SCHIP), and health insurance portability standards.

CPOE Computerized Physician (or Provider) Order Entry
The process of electronic entry of medical practitioner instructions for the treatment of patients.

CQM Clinical Quality Measures
The processes, experience, and/or outcomes of patient care, observations, or treatment that relate to one or more quality aims for health care such as effective, safe, efficient, patient-centered, equitable, and timely care. Under the current CMS EHR Incentive Programs there are 44 CQMs in total.

EH Eligible Hospital
The designation provided to hospitals that meet certain criteria under the CMS EHR Incentive Programs.

EHR Electronic Health Record
A systematic collection of electronic health information about individual patients or populations.

EMR Electronic Medical Record
A computerized medical record created in an organization that delivers care, such as a hospital or physician's office.

EP Eligible Professional
The designation provided to individual physicians that meet certain criteria under the CMS EHR Incentive Programs.

FACA Federal Advisory Committee Act
A United States law which governs the behavior of federal advisory committees by restricting the formation of such committees to only those which are deemed essential, limits their powers to provision of advice to officers and agencies in the executive branch of the Federal Government, and limits the length of term during which any such committee may operate.

FFS Fee-for-Service
Payment model where services are unbundled and paid for separately. In health care, it gives an incentive for physicians to provide more treatments because payment is dependent on the quantity of care, rather than quality of care.

HHS U.S. Department of Health and Human Services
A Cabinet department of the United States government with the goal of protecting the health of all Americans and providing essential human services.

HIE Health Information Exchange
The mobilization of healthcare information electronically across organizations within a region, community, or hospital system.

HIPAA Health Insurance Portability and Accountability Act
Enacted in 1996, HIPAA protects health insurance coverage for workers and their families when they change or lose their jobs and requires the establishment of national standards for electronic health care transactions and national identifiers for providers, health insurance plans, and employers.

HIT Health Information Technology
Umbrella framework to describe the comprehensive management of health information across computerized systems and its secure exchange between consumers, providers, government and quality entities, and insurers.

HITECH Health Information Technology for Economic and Clinical Health
Enacted as part of the American Recovery and Reinvestment Act of 2009, it promotes the adoption and meaningful use of health information technology.

HITRC Healthcare Information Technology Research Center
Helps RECs work with one another and with relevant stakeholders to identify and share best practices in EHR adoption, meaningful use, and provider support.

HITSP Healthcare Information Technology Standards Panel
A cooperative partnership between the public and private sectors for the purpose of promoting interoperability in health care by harmonizing health information technology standards.

HL7 Health Level Seven
An all-volunteer, non-profit organization involved in development of international healthcare informatics interoperability standards.

HPSA Health Professional Shortage Area
Identifies areas of greater need for health care services in order to direct limited health care professional resources to people in those areas. There are currently more than six thousand shortage areas.

ICD International Classification for Diseases
A medical classification that provides codes to classify diseases and a wide variety of signs, symptoms, abnormal findings, complaints, social circumstances, and external causes of injury or disease.

NIST National Institute of Standards and Technology
A measurement standards laboratory, which is a non-regulatory agency of the United States Department of Commerce, dedicated to promoting U.S. innovation and industrial competitiveness by advancing measurement science, standards, and technology in ways that enhance economic security and improve our quality of life.

NLM National Library of Medicine
Operated by the United States Federal Government, it is the world's largest medical library with more than seven million books, journals, technical reports, manuscripts, photographs, and images on medicine and related sciences.

NPI National Provider Identifier
A unique 10-digit identification number issued to health care providers in the United States by the Centers for Medicare and Medicaid Services.

NPPES National Plan and Provider Enumeration System
Standard unique identifiers for health care providers and health plans provisioned by the Health Insurance Portability and Accountability Act of 1996.

NPRM Notice of Proposed Rulemaking
A public notice issued by law when one of the independent agencies of the United States government wishes to add, remove, or change a rule or regulation as part of the rulemaking process.

NQF National Quality Forum
A nonprofit organization that is dedicated to improving the quality of health care in the United States.

ONC Office of National Coordinator for Health Information Technology
A staff division of the Office of the Secretary, within the U.S. Department of Health and Human Services, that is primarily focused on coordination of nationwide efforts to implement and use health information technology and the electronic exchange of health information.

PECOS Provider Enrollment, Chain, and Ownership System
The Internet-based system can be used in lieu of the Medicare enrollment application to submit an initial Medicare enrollment application, view or change enrollment information, track an enrollment application through the web submission process, add or change a reassignment of benefits, submit changes to existing Medicare enrollment information, reactivate an existing enrollment record, and withdraw from the Medicare Program.

PQRI Physician Quality Reporting Initiative
Provides incentive payments to eligible physicians and other practitioners who adequately report data on quality measures for covered services furnished during a given reporting period.

REC Regional Extension Center
Regional centers that were created to support and serve health care providers and help them quickly become adept and meaningful users of electronic health records.

XML Extensible Markup Language
A set of rules for encoding documents in machine-readable form.

Appendix

Sources

American College of Radiology. Government Relations. Meaningful Use Resources. Web. < http://www.acr.org/SecondaryMainMenuCategories/GR_Econ/Meaningful-Use-Resource-Center.aspx/>.

U.S. Department of Commerce. The National Institute of Standards and Technology. Health Information Technology. Standards and Testing. Meaningful Use Test Method. Web. <http://www.nist.gov/healthcare/testing/mutestmethod.cfm/>.

U.S. Department of Health and Human Services. Centers for Medicare & Medicaid Services. CMS EHR Incentive Programs Official Website. Web. <http://www.cms.gov/ehrincentiveprograms/>.

U.S. Department of Health and Human Services. Centers for Medicare & Medicaid Services. Medicare and Medicaid Programs; Electronic Health Record Incentive Program. Comparison of Meaningful Use Objectives Between the Proposed Rule to the Final Rule. 13 July 2010. Web.

U.S. Department of Health and Human Services. Centers for Medicare & Medicaid Services. Medicare and Medicaid Programs; Electronic Health Record Incentive Program. Final Rule. 42 CFR Parts 412, 413, 422, and 495. 28 July 2010. Print.

U.S. Department of Health and Human Services. Office of the National Coordinator for Health Information Technology. Establishment of the Temporary Certification Program for Health Information Technology. Part II. Final Rule. 42 CFR Parts 170. 24 June 2010. Print.

U.S. Department of Health and Human Services. Office of the National Coordinator for Health Information Technology. Federal Advisory Committee Blog. Web. <http://healthit.hhs.gov/blog/faca/>.

U.S. Department of Health and Human Services. Office of the National Coordinator for Health Information Technology. Health Information Technology: Initial Set of Standards, Implementation Specifications, and Certification Criteria for Electronic Health Record Technology. Part III. Final Rule. 42 CFR Parts 170. 28 July 2010. Print.

U.S. Department of Health and Human Services. Office of the National Coordinator for Health Information Technology. Health Information Technology: Initial Set of Standards, Implementation Specifications, and Certification Criteria for Electronic Health Record Technology. Interim Final Rule. 42 CFR Parts 170. 13 January 2010. Print.

U.S. Department of Health and Human Services. Office of the National Coordinator for Health Information Technology. HealthITBuzz Blog. Web. <http://www.healthit.gov/buzz-blog/>.

U.S. Department of Health and Human Services. Office of the National Coordinator for Health Information Technology. Regulations and Guidance. Electronic Health Records and Meaningful Use. Web. <http://healthit.hhs.gov/portal/server.pt?open=512&objID=2996&mode=2>.

Index

$44,000, **10, 22, 24, 40-43, 219**

10 Menu Set, **24-25, 48, 52, 219**

15 Core Set, **24-25, 48-49, 219**

25 Objectives and Measures, **34, 109**

33 Certification Criteria, **34, 65, 87, 97**

44 Clinical Quality Measures, **24-25, 48, 56**

A

ABR, **31, 158, 191, 211**

ACR, **31-32, 104, 107, 190-192, 211**

Adjustments, **24, 42, 105, 170, 205, 218**

ARRA, **14, 30-32, 70, 82, 105, 175, 190, 218, 226**

Ascension Path, **35**

Attestation, **43, 118, 122, 133, 144-151, 217, 220-221**

Audit, **73, 85, 112, 133, 151, 221**

B

Blog, **107**

C

Calculator, **147, 221**

CCHIT, **32, 82, 84**

Certification Criteria, **31, 65, 70-81, 85-87, 97, 190**

CFR, **48-55, 65, 71-81, 95-96, 110-111, 149,151, 226**

Challenges, **92, 96-97**

CHPL, **87, 106, 134, 147, 226**

Classification, **23-24, 40, 110, 112**

Clinical Quality Measures, **24-25, 48, 50, 56, 76, 78, 80, 111, 227**

CMS Final Rule, **32, 35, 151, 219**

Complete EHR, **82, 85, 123, 137-138**

Continuing Extension Act, **23, 31-32, 107**

Core Set, **25, 43, 48-52, 110, 147**

D

Dashboards, **146, 161, 170, 185**

Dates, **205**

Denominators, **43, 95, 148, 170, 221**

Discretionary, **56-59**

Drummond Group, **32, 82, 84**

E

Eligibility, **23, 107-108, 119, 159, 167, 176, 182, 217**

Exclusions, **49-55, 109, 148**

Exemptions, **42, 52, 56**

F

FACA, **32, 227**

Fact Sheets, **106**

FAQ, **86, 94-95, 216-221**

Financial Impact, **93, 107-108, 159, 167, 176, 182**

G

Goals, **23**

H

HHS, **32, 64, 70, 82, 227**

HIE, **227**

HITECH, **22-23, 30-31, 34, 228**

HPSA, **41, 43, 228**

I

ICSA Labs, **32, 83**

IFR, **31**

Imaging EMR, **92, 169**

Implementation, **133-138**

Incentive Payment, **41-43, 105, 145, 148, 205, 218**

Incentives, **30, 218**

Infogard Laboratories, **32, 83-84**

L

Legislation, **30-33, 42, 70, 105**

Listserv, **204**

M

Medicaid EHR Incentive Program, **35, 86, 94-95, 108**

Medicare EHR Incentive Program, **35, 86, 94-95, 107-109, 219**

Menu Set, **25, 52-56, 111, 149-151**

Modular EHR, **79, 85**

Monitoring, **146, 161, 170, 178-179, 185**

Multiple Locations, **93, 176**

N

NIST, **70-81, 86, 228**

NPI, **144-145, 229**

NPPES, **144, 229**

NPRM, **31, 229**

NQF, **57-59, 111-112, 229**

Numerators, **43, 50, 56, 73, 146, 148**

O

ONC-ATCB, **65, 70, 79, 82, 84, 86, 124**

ONC Final Rule, **32-33, 86**

P

PECOS, **144, 229**

Penalties, **42, 93, 218**

POS, **23-24, 49, 95, 107**

Possess, **85-86, 93, 97, 123, 219**

Practice Analyzer, **104, 110, 159**

Q

QR Codes, **16, 21, 29, 39, 47, 63, 69, 91, 103, 117, 131, 143, 189, 197, 209, 215, 225**

Questions, **107-110, 124-125, 133, 159**

R

REC, **148, 199-204, 229**

Record Keeping, **151**

Registration, **144-145, 161, 170, 178, 185, 221**

Regulations, **33-35, 87, 210-11**

Reporting Period, **40, 94-95, 147-148**

Requirements, **34-35, 48-49, 93, 149-151**

Resources, **104-107, 198-204**

RSNA, **31-32, 191, 211**

S

Seen by the EP, **94-96**

SIIM, **31, 191, 211**

SLI Global Solutions, **32, 83-84**

Stage 1, **22, 24, 35, 48, 92, 210**

Stage 2, **25, 35, 191-192, 205, 210**

Stage 3, **25, 35, 205, 210-211**

Stakeholders, **118, 160, 168, 176, 183**

Surescripts, **32, 83-84**

T

Taskforce, **120-122, 168-169**

TIN, **145, 219**

V

Vendors, **65, 92, 123-127**

About the authors

Jonathon L. Dreyer is a senior health care marketing professional in Boston, Massachusetts. His deep understanding of medical imaging technology and healthcare IT has contributed to the development and successful deployment of technology across a number of health care verticals. He has authored several articles on clinical decision support, radiology reporting, speech recognition, business intelligence, electronic health records, meaningful use, and mHealth, and is an active blogger and contributor to standards and interoperability projects.

Keith J. Dreyer, DO, PhD, FSIIM is the Vice Chairman of Radiology Informatics at Massachusetts General Hospital and Assistant Professor of Radiology at the Harvard Medical School. He is a Diagnostic Radiologist, certified by the American Board of Radiology with a PhD in Computer Science. Dr. Dreyer holds, and has held, numerous board and committee positions with the ACR, RSNA, SIIM, and other national medical societies, and has authored numerous scientific papers, articles, and books, as well as lectures worldwide on digital imaging, medical informatics, clinical language understanding, and electronic health records.

Made in the USA
Monee, IL
07 July 2026

56552168R00134